THE NEW
W.E.T. Workout®

THE NEW
W.E.T. Workout®

Water Exercise Techniques for Strengthening, Toning, and Lifetime Fitness

JANE KATZ, ED.D.

☑® Facts On File, Inc.

AN INFOBASE HOLDINGS COMPANY

Facts On File, Inc.
11 Penn Plaza
New York, NY 10001

Library of Congress Cataloging-in-Publication Data

Katz, Jane.
    The new W.E.T. workout : water exercise techniques for strengthening, toning, and lifetime fitness / Jane Katz.
        p. cm.
    Includes index.
    ISBN 0-8160-3268-8 (hbk.). — ISBN 0-8160-3342-0 (pbk.)
    1. Aquatic exercises. I. Title.
RA781.17.K376 1996
613.7'16—dc20   95-48450

Facts On File books are available at special discounts when purchased in bulk quantities for businesses, associations, institutions or sales promotions. Please call our Special Sales Department in New York at 212/967-8800 or 800/322-8755.

Text design by Catherine Rincon Hyman
Cover design by Matt Galemmo
Illustrations by Dale Dyer and Ann Jasperson

The W.E.T. Workout® is a registered trademark of Jane Katz, Ed.D.

This book is printed on acid-free paper.

Printed in the United States of America

RRD FOF 10 9 8 7 6 5 4 3 2 1

Photo Credits:

Front cover: Members of the National Fitness Assn. Courtesy of Ebel Photography International

Back cover photograph courtesy of Speedo® Authentic Fitness

Page iv: Fran Vogel
Pages 16–17: Courtesy Diagram
Page 10: *Sports Illustrated*
Page 79: Speedo® Authentic Fitness
Page 86: Speedo® Authentic Fitness
Page 104: Aroldo Macedo
Page 134: Patricia Berland
Page 145: Daniel Kron
Page 155: ICI Acrylic
Page 166: Endless Pools
Page 170: Col. Willie Davenport
Page 182: Shane Neumark

This book is dedicated to

water lovers everywhere,

as we plunge

into the new millennium.

Contents

Foreword

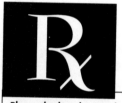

Jane Katz, Ed. D., has written *The New W.E.T. Workout*® for all those who enjoy being in the water (and for those who think they might). Virtually everyone will benefit from utilizing this instructive book.

Water has major advantages as an exercise medium, due largely to two important, helpful forces: *buoyancy* and *resistance*.

❑ A person in the water displaces a volume of water, resulting in an upward lifting force (buoyancy) that allows an individual to do less work against the downward pull of gravity, freeing up energy that can be used to overcome the resistance of water.

❑ The faster one moves through the water, the more resistance is created. Consequently, muscles are strengthened.

❑ There is a comfort zone that is different for everyone. Working within this comfort zone makes it possible for everyone to participate, from people in peak condition to those with special needs. Age is no limitation.

❑ Better muscular and cardiovascular conditioning is made possible with greater safety by doing *The New W.E.T. Workout.*® People exercising in the water can reach a certain level of exertion with a smaller increase in heart rate than would occur when exercising on land.

❑ People with musculoskeletal concerns (such as sports-related injuries or arthritis) appear to suffer less pain and become more mobile in water than on land. Increasingly, health professionals, in their quest to promote good health and prevent (or heal) injuries, are now recommending the inclusion of water exercises to allow people of all shapes, sizes and disabilities to recondition themselves.

This book is invaluable for all who aim to develop good health in a conducive environment, so that muscular and cardiovascular fitness are maintained.

Herbert L. Erlanger, MD
Attending Anesthesiologist
New York Hospital,
Cornell Medical Center

The New W.E.T. World

The W.E.T. Workout® was borne out of adversity. I had sustained severe injuries as a result of a car accident caused by a drunk driver. At the time, sports medicine as a specialty was in its infancy. Just obtaining a waterproof cast for my fractured wrist was virtually impossible. I improvised a covering from plastic grocery bags, and continued my recovery by creating Water Exercise Techniques. This was the foundation of *The W.E.T. Workout*® program for general wellness, which was published in 1985. It appeared at a time when the benefits of exercise were just beginning to become widely recognized by the general public. It was some fifteen years after the phrase "aerobic exercise" was coined by Dr. Kenneth Cooper to describe any physical activity that improves the body's capacity to bring in oxygen and deliver it to tissue cells to produce energy. Many people were beginning exercise programs for the first time in their adult lives to take advantage of the benefits: increased strength and muscle tone, improved appearance, weight control, and the positive correlation between sustained physical activity and cardiovascular health. Medical studies were indicating the positive effect of exercise on overall health as well as psychological well-being. This ongoing research continues to confirm that physical fitness should be a way of life, as stated by the *Surgeon General's Report on Physical Activity and Health*.

The W.E.T. Workout program appeared as one of a number of programs promising improved fitness. However, as the exercise boom of the 1970s and 1980s peaked, and the baby-boom generation matured, a growing need for moderation in fitness choices became evident. The "healthiest" people were beginning to complain of aches and pains. A major concern was high-impact injuries: The jumping and jogging was more than many mature bodies could sustain. What was needed was a fitness activity that would combine stretching, aerobic conditioning,

> "The Surgeon General has determined that lack of physical activity is detrimental to your health."

strength training, and flexibility. Exercising in water was the answer.

Then there was the other half of the American population that did not swim well enough to get an aerobic workout, had never learned to swim, or had had a bad experience in or near the water, and were afraid. Among them were also people who didn't swim for such reasons as, "I can swim but I can't breathe," "I don't want to get my hair wet," or "I'm overweight and I'm embarrassed to be seen exercising." For these people The W.E.T. Workout offered an ideal fitness activity by adapting land exercises to the water. There was a burgeoning of water exercise classes, variously labeled hydro-calisthenics, hydro-slimnastics, aquarobics or aquacise. Today, they are the staple of aquatic fitness programs at Ys, community pools, and health clubs throughout the country. Approximately seven million people in the U.S. now participate in some form of water exercise. (This is in addition to the millions who continue to swim laps for fitness.)

As water exercise has developed, so have the varieties of ways to exercise in water, as has the state-of-the-art equipment and the sophistication of its adherents. Many types of water exercise classes have become extremely popular.

The New W.E.T. Workout is designed to reflect the developments in water exercise. For instance, it has expanded into the areas of sports cross-training, prescriptive therapy, pregnancy fitness, swimming and synchronized swimming starters, and family fun. One of the qualities of the original W.E.T. Workout program is its simplicity. This new edition aims to maintain that particular approach. I hope you enjoy *The New W.E.T. Workout*® well into the twenty-first century!

Jane Katz, Ed. D.
New York City

Acknowledgments

On a personal note, I have understood and experienced the magic of water for wellness. I and many of my aquatic colleagues have been in the vanguard of the movement to make this a popular fitness activity available to everyone. Supporting me in this endeavor, and my special thanks to them, are:

My parents—Dorothea and Leon, who introduced me to the wonders of water fun.

My sisters and brother—June Guzman, Paul Katz, and Elaine Kuperberg, and their children Jason, Justin, Austen, Autumn, and Stephen, for our time enjoying and playing in the water together.

To Elaine Fincham, Charlet Oberley, and Elaine Kuperberg for helping in all phases of this new splash.

For Jason Guzman and Ann Jasperson whose initial illustrations highlighted the enjoyment of Water Exercise Techniques, and especially to Dale Dyer.

I'd especially like to thank Herbert L. Erlanger, M.D., for his unswerving support and timely foreword.

Many thanks to the Facts On File staff who helped produce this book—Beverly Balaz, Andrea Brown, Andrew Galli, Josh Karpf, Mark McDonnell, Hilary Poole, Tim Reynolds, Catherine Rincon, and particularly Jeffrey Golick, Emily Ross, Laurie Likoff, and Phil Saltz.

To the many aquatic specialists who have been supportive of *The W.E.T. Workout*® program. And a salute to the aquatic industry for its commitment to water fitness.

Finally, thanks to all the water lovers everywhere who have enjoyed W.E.T. workouts everywhere.

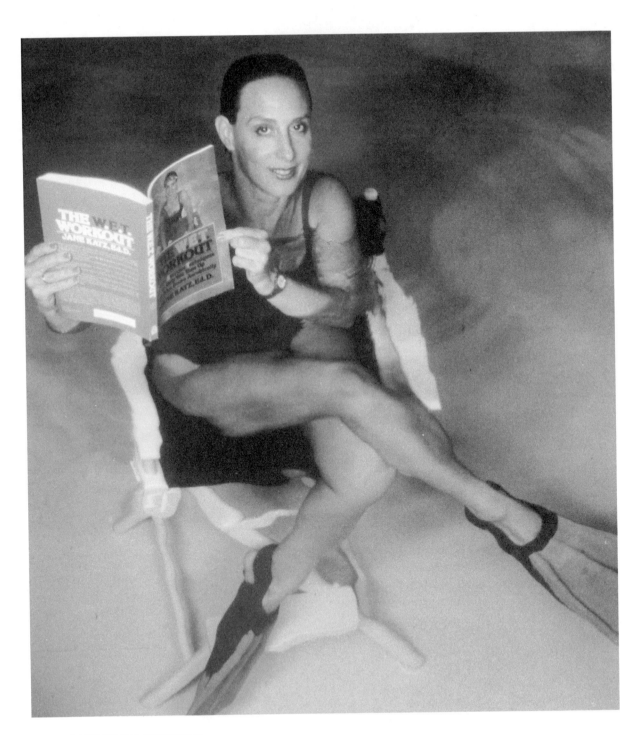

Introduction to Water Exercise Techniques

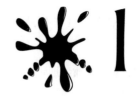

Water! It's the perfect environment for exercising, losing weight, strengthening and toning muscles, reducing stress, relaxing, and simply having fun! Water allows you to get the most out of an exercise program. Simply put, water works! Exercising in water helps you gain the many benefits of exercise enjoyably and without stress or pain.

Many types of exercises will help make you fit. But let's face it: Not all of them are enjoyable. All exercise requires a certain amount of effort—but effort is different from discomfort. You can enjoy exercising in water with *The New W.E.T. Workout.*® And if you enjoy your exercise program, you have a much better chance of staying with it—and reaping the benefits.

This program includes a workout for everyone—from challenging *Water Exercise Techniques* (hence, W.E.T.s) for the energetic, to relaxed programs for those who prefer a less vigorous routine. For those of you who are short on time, I've included exercises you can do during your lunch hour, without even getting your hair wet. For those of you with music in your soul, there are exercises adapted from synchronized swimming. No matter what your choice, in *The New W.E.T. Workout*® you'll find an exercise program that will leave you refreshed, not fatigued; exhilarated, not exhausted. You'll improve your aerobic capacity, strength, and flexibility, and it can even help you lose weight!

In 1896 the first Olympic Games of modern times were held in Athens, Greece, with the swimming competitions taking place in open water. In the same year halfway across the world in San Francisco, the Sutro Baths were opened to the public. They provided a choice of seven pools of varying size and temperatures, six of which had ocean water and one fresh water.

The Sutro Baths were called "the Coney Island of the West." They were considered a pleasure palace for the entire family—a forerunner of today's recreational water parks.

This spectacular facility was designed and built by Adolph Sutro, an engineer and proponent of physical exercise for the public. He "always held swimming to be the very best exercise."

Benefits and Properties of Water

Water, water, everywhere . . .

Most of the earth is composed of water. There's water surrounding us all the time. It's part of every living thing. Two-thirds of our bodies are made up of water. Many of our leisure pursuits take place in and around water (just check the travel section of any newspaper and note the photos). People have long taken advantage of water's relaxing and healing properties. The Romans were famous for their baths, as are now the Japanese. Popular natural mineral springs at Spa, Belgium, added a new word to our language. In the eighteenth and nineteenth centuries, hydropathy, the use of water in the treatment of injury and illness, became very popular. Hydrotherapists used cold water to reduce swelling caused by strains and sprains and to decrease fevers, and warm water to increase blood circulation and to calm patients. Many of the concepts of hydrotherapy are widely used today in modern physical therapy. For example, today's physical therapists use underwater exercises to help patients strengthen weakened muscles, to help them relax torn and strained muscles, and to improve muscle function in patients recovering from strokes and injuries. Warm-water massages (whirlpool spas) are often used to help heal injuries and to promote relaxation.

Water, this "magic medium," is what makes The New W.E.T. Workout® program different from land exercise regimens. As you ease yourself into the water, the day's tensions ebb away. The relaxation eases your mind and strengthens your body. The water keeps you cool even when you exercise.

The buoyancy of the water allows your body to feel almost weightless. In chin-deep water, your apparent weight is one tenth of your true weight on land. The water supports you, adding grace and fluidity to your movements. This natural phenomenon allows your muscles, joints, and ligaments to move freely and comfortably without pounding, straining, or jarring. Also, exercising in water helps increase joint flexibility, which is a special advantage for those with arthritis.

Water provides a natural resistance because it is twelve times denser than air. This means that when you are exercising in water your muscles have to work harder than in air. You see the results of your exercise faster in terms of increased strength and better muscle tone.

Water will help support, heal, and relax muscles that may be strained or tightened by other activities. For sports injuries, W.E.T. workouts can help you recover quickly and return to your former level of fitness.

Join the W.E.T. Set

A quick check of the local "health clubs" will probably prove quite rewarding in finding facilities. Don't forget to check for local Ys. You may also find that community centers and schools have pools open to the public; most large hotels, and many smaller ones, have swimming facilities available to guests and to the public. Unless you're tripping off to a desert, you should be able to find a place to do your W.E.T. workouts—you can do them in lakes, ponds, and rivers, and on beaches, too. Don't let the weather put a damper on your program. In much of the world the summer is too short, so don't be afraid to do your W.E.T. workout indoors for much of the year. And best yet, you can do W.E.T. workouts privately if you're fortunate enough to have your own backyard pool, no matter what its size or shape.

The W.E.T. exercises I describe can be used by everyone. No matter what your age or physical condition, this book offers you a program that will help you look and feel terrific. Since the program is progressive, you can get started without undue stress and strain, then gradually improve your level of fitness and maintain it.

Improved aerobic capacity, flexibility, and strength are only the most obvious benefits you will derive from this program. Recent medical evidence has demonstrated that people who are physically fit are:

    able to keep their weight under control
    sick less often
    healthier in their outlook on life
    less tense
    younger looking
    able to handle stress better

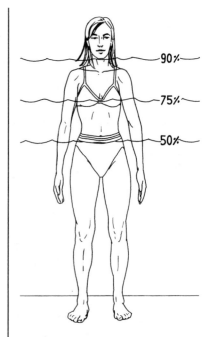

About Aerobic Exercise

What exactly are aerobic exercises? Those that benefit your cardiovascular system. Your cardiovascular system carries blood to your working muscles, supplying them with oxygen from the air you breathe and eliminating carbon dioxide and other waste products. Your ability to accomplish these biological tasks is called your "aerobic capacity." The stronger and more efficient your heart and lungs, the greater your aerobic capacity. The greater your aerobic capacity, the less strain on your heart, the greater your ability to perform work, the greater your ability to cope with stress, and the greater your feeling of well-being.

One of the most important goals in being physically fit is improving your aerobic capacity. No matter how big your biceps, without a strong cardiovascular system, you are not truly fit. In addition, there are other components of physical fitness that are enhanced by your new W.E.T. workout: improved endurance, greater coordination and strength, an increased range of motion, flexibility, agility, balance, and a kinesthetic awareness.

Anatomy of a Workout

A water fitness workout should include the key elements of any workout: a warm-up, the main set, and a cool-down for a total workout time of 20–45 minutes.

The *warm-up* is a five-minute period during which the water exerciser prepares the muscles and the cardiovascular system for work by slowly loosening and stretching the muscles, and elevating the heart rate. This period enables the exerciser to adjust from a land environment to water.

The *main set* is the aerobic part of the workout, consisting of 20 to 30 minutes of continuous movement in the water designed to exercise all areas of the body while accelerating the pulse to its target heart rate (THR).

The *cool-down* concludes the workout with approximately five minutes of easy stretches and relaxation exercises to gradually return the body to its warm-up state and heart rate.

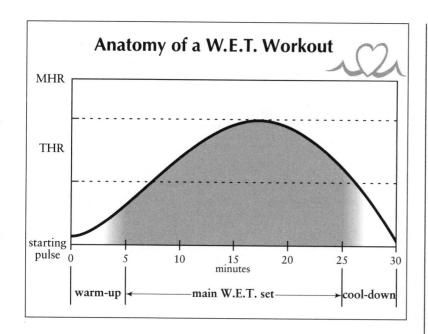

Anatomy of a W.E.T. Workout

MHR

THR

starting pulse

0   5   10   15   20   25   30
minutes

warm-up | main W.E.T. set | cool-down

Target Heart Rate

There are several ways to check how aerobically you are doing your W.E.T. workout. A common method of measuring the aerobic effectiveness of your workout is checking your pulse rate at various points and comparing them to each other at various phases. Your pulse rate at the beginning of your workout should be lower than during your main set. To find your target heart rate (THR), the rate to which you want to gear your workout, both the American Heart Association and the American Medical Association recommend the following formula, which first calculates your maximum heart rate (MHR), based on your age. The MHR is 220 minus your chronological age. So if a person is 45, his or her MHR is 175 beats per minute (bpm).

The target heart rate or THR for this person's workout should be about between 60% to 80% of the MHR, depending on your fitness level and the intensity of the workout. In this case the THR would be 105 to 140. If you are 20 years of age, the target heart rate range would be 120 to 160 ((220–20) x 60% to 80%).

To calculate your heart rate, take your pulse at either wrist or on either side of your neck at the carotid artery. Hold a finger on

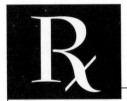

For those who wish to or need to monitor their heart rate throughout their W.E.T. workout, waterproof heart rate monitors are available.

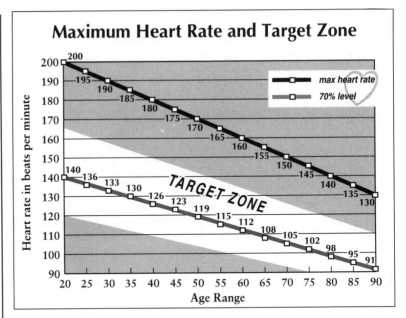

Maximum Heart Rate and Target Zone

the pulse and count the number of beats for six seconds. Multiply the number of beats by 10 by adding a 0.

Take your pulse at the beginning of the warm-up, during your main set, and during your cool-down. Use the figures to check the intensity of your workout.

Perceived Energy Exertion

Researchers in exercise physiology have found that exercisers themselves are best able to provide an accurate guide to how hard they are really working.

As exercisers increase exertion, their heart rates rise in proportion to the increase in effort. Exercisers working below their target heart rate (based on pulse count) perceive that their energy exertion is light to moderate. As exercisers approach maximum heart rate, their perceived energy exertion is at a very high level.

Use the table below as a guide for perceived energy exertion. Correlate perceived energy exertion with the number in the left column. Then compare your perceived exertion to your target heart rate (THR) range.

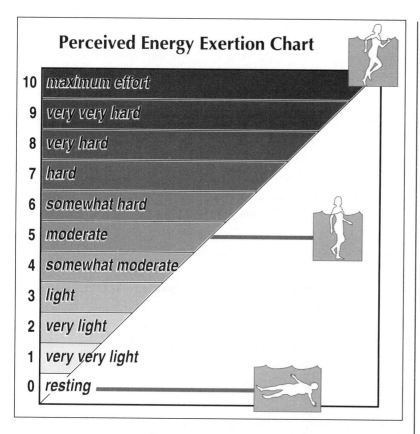

Perceived Energy Exertion Chart

10	maximum effort
9	very very hard
8	very hard
7	hard
6	somewhat hard
5	moderate
4	somewhat moderate
3	light
2	very light
1	very very light
0	resting

With increased physical conditioning, the resting heart rate becomes lower than it was in the pre-fitness state because the heart is stronger and is working more efficiently.

Talk Test

A simple guideline for perceived energy exertion is the talk test. If you can carry on a conversation while exercising, you are probably not overexerting yourself. However, if you are not able to talk, you are most likely approaching your maximum exertion level and maximum target heart rate for your age. A unique benefit of participating in water exercise is that your body can be submerged in water while your face remains out of the water. Therefore, you can easily monitor your perceived energy exertion by applying the talk test.

SAFETY TIPS

A water fitness program is best enjoyed if you follow basic guidelines for safety and courtesy.

☐ **Get a medical checkup before beginning this or any exercise program.** This is especially important if you are beginning an exercise program after being sedentary (like a couch potato).

☐ Safety comes first. Exercise with supervision. **Never exercise alone.**

☐ **Check the depth of the water before going in;** enter the pool in shallow water.

☐ **When entering the water,** sit on the deck with both hands on the same side of your body. Turn your body toward your hands as you slowly lower your body to a standing position, in the pool, facing the wall.

☐ **Start slowly and listen to your body.** Water exercise doesn't "feel" strenuous, so it is easy to do too much too soon. Pace your workouts, and rest when you need to.

☐ Breathe rhythmically and continuously. **Never hold your breath!**

☐ It is important to **hydrate** both before and after exercising. Water is best!

☐ Always **warm up** before your main W.E.T. set and **cool down** afterward.

☐ **If pain, shortness of breath, dizziness, or disorientation** occur during exercise, **stop,** leave the water, and rest.

☐ Have **fun**. Take the plunge!

F.I.T. Principle

To achieve an aerobic training effect, overload the body progressively by increasing the *F*requency, *I*ntensity, and *T*ime of the workout. The main set is the central part of the workout where this F.I.T. principle is applied which includes exercises for the upper, middle, lower, and total body. (See page 53.)

So suit up and take the plunge into the exhilarating world of W.E.T. workouts!

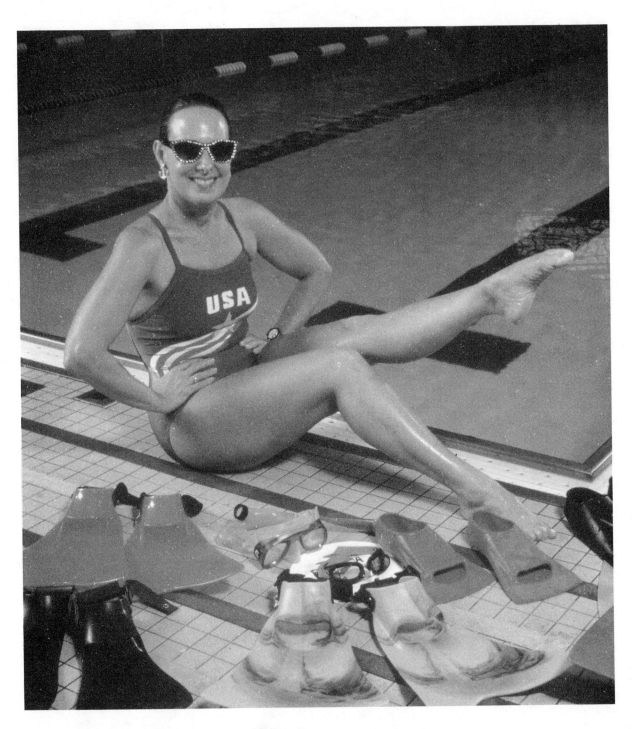

The Basic Water Exercise Techniques Program

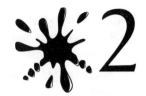

Getting Started: Gearing Up

Before you take the W.E.T. plunge, you'll need to gear up with just a few items.

Your Personal Musts

Swimsuit. A stretch Lycra suit is light, quick drying, and very comfortable. Lycra body suits (with shorts attached) are also available.

My motto is don't leave home without your swimsuit. Then you can do W.E.T. workouts anywhere!

Pace clock or waterproof wristwatch. Give each exercise portion and each workout session its full, allotted time. You will need a waterproof watch or a pace clock usually available poolside to keep tabs on your time. Don't cheat yourself.

Aqua shoes. Waterproof shoes usually made of nylon mesh with a rubberlike sole. They are helpful for cushioning feet during water exercise as well as protecting feet and providing traction on a pool deck. They are highly recommended.

Optional

Swim cap. If you're concerned about keeping your hair dry and protecting it, use a latex (rubber) cap.

If you prefer an easy-to-pull-on cap, or if you have long hair, a Lycra (stretch) cap can be better. There are other materials and caps available, such as a silicone-based rubber cap.

Goggles. If you wear contact lenses or are sensitive to chemically treated water or salt water, you should use a pair of goggles. In addition to protecting your eyes, goggles allow you to see clearly underwater. It's a whole new universe!

Aquatic Equipment

Kickboard. A kickboard is a flotation device that supports the upper body, allowing swimmers to practice kicks. It also can be used as a resistance device.

Hand paddles, mitts, and gloves. Paddles are resistance devices for the upper body. Placed on your hands, they offer greater resistance to the water. They're like fins for your hands. Try hand paddles when you perform upper-body W.E.T.s such as the medley of strokes (see page 29). Mitts and gloves are also worn on the hands, with the larger surface area increasing resistance during arm motion, and enhancing arm and shoulder exercises.

Pull-buoy. A pull-buoy is a small float, usually made of styrofoam. It is often used by swimmers to support the lower body. A pull-buoy can be used both as a flotation device (placed behind the neck of a back floater) and as a resistance device during certain exercises.

Fins. Fins are large paddles that attach to the feet. There are many different weights, shapes, and styles. Commonly used for skin diving, they offer excellent propulsion and help to increase flexibility, strength, and speed. Use them for variety when performing lower leg W.E.T.s.

Cuffs. These are flotation/resistance devices (sometimes inflatable) that can be placed on the arms or legs. They can be used as a flotation device for easy, relaxed floating and/or as a resistance device.

Flotation belts and/or vests. Belts made of styrofoam or other buoyant material keep the exerciser's head just above water. They are made of a thin buoyant lightweight material to provide neutral buoyancy without bulkiness. These are ideal for deep-water exercise, e.g., deep-water running.

Barbells. These are flotation devices shaped as the name implies. They are also available in molded plastic which offers greater resistance, rather than buoyancy.

Aqua step. A step similar to an aerobic step that is designed to be used in a pool. The additional height of the step offers a wide variety of exercise possibilities.

Tethered exercise. These are exercises in which the swimmer is usually attached to the side of the pool by a stretch cord in order to practice against its resistance. There are also variations, such as a "chute" for increased resistance.

Logs. Logs are solid Styrofoam tubes approximately five feet long and three inches in diameter. They are buoyant, flexible, versatile, and fun! They are sometimes also called *noodles*.

See chapter 4 for specific W.E.T. equipment exercises.

Large Equipment

Spas. A water tank in which water jets concentrate the flow of water to create resistance; workouts using jets allow for greater effort and can provide relaxation benefits.

Jets. Water jets in spas are often used for intensified water-massaging action on various body parts such as the ankle, knee, shoulder and wrist joints, and back.

Water treadmill. Similar to a walking treadmill, it is placed in the water so the exerciser can actively walk/jog in chin- to chest-deep water.

Water workout stations. Multipurpose equipment machinery placed in the pool against pool wall.

The above are sample highlights of aquatic exercise available. As the trend to exercise in water continues to expand, additional water exercise equipment will become available for the aquatic market.

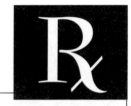

PERSONAL SAFETY CHECK

Check with your doctor before starting W.E.T.s, especially if you've recently been under a physician's care.

Listen to your body. If you experience any significant discomfort or pain, ease up on your exercises; if the problem persists, see your doctor.

Check the water depth and pool layout before you begin. Be certain that your swimming facility is supervised properly. There should always be a lifeguard on duty.

Tips for Group Participation

Have more fun in the water by exercising with a group, with friends and swim buddies, or in a class situation. Here are some suggestions for group W.E.T. exercise.

Four or more people in the water: make a circle.

Do synchronized swimming exercises: swim in a pattern, such as a Christmas tree.

For a large group, exercise in two lines, and change sides as part of your exercise routine.

Some safety tips to be aware of:

❑ Position taller people in deeper water
❑ Position overweight people in shallower water
❑ Those who need help in balancing should exercise near the wall or corner of the pool
❑ When proceeding from one exercise to the next, do a "shake out" (see page 50)
❑ For best comfort in shallow water, exercise in chin- to chest-deep water

Warm-Ups and Cool-Downs

Before each workout, you need to warm up; after each water workout, you need to cool-down. Each warm-up and cool-down should last approximately five minutes. Warm-ups are essential because your body, especially the muscles, needs time to gear up, stretch, and get ready for action. If you skip your warm up, you're more likely to strain a muscle or injure a joint. Cooling down and stretching out after your workout helps you to relax, cool off, and bring your body back to its normal state.

Some of the warm-ups and cool downs included are standard exercises incorporated into most workouts. An important type of warm-up and cool-down exercise is a slow and progressive stretch: one in which you reach your maximum comfortable extension and hold for approximately 30 seconds. Remember that stretching should always be a slow and steady movement rather than a sharp and forced one.

Body Areas

The W.E.T.s in this book benefit all body areas and muscle groups:

Upper Body

- ❏ head and neck (sternocleidomastoid)
- ❏ wrist, hand grip, and forearm (pronators)
- ❏ upper arm and back of arm (biceps and triceps)
- ❏ shoulders (deltoids)
- ❏ chest (pectorals)
- ❏ upper back (trapezius and latissimus dorsi)

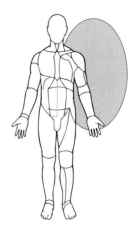

Middle Body

- ❏ sides of trunk
- ❏ middle back
- ❏ rib cage (intercostals)
- ❏ waist (abdominals)
- ❏ lower back
- ❏ pelvic area

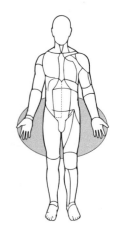

Lower Body

- ❏ thighs (hamstrings—back of thighs, quadriceps—front of thighs)
- ❏ groin, inner thigh (sartorius)
- ❏ buttocks (gluteus maximus)
- ❏ hips
- ❏ calves (gastrocnemius—back)
- ❏ knees
- ❏ ankle and foot (Achilles tendon)

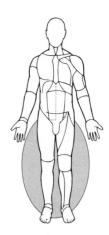

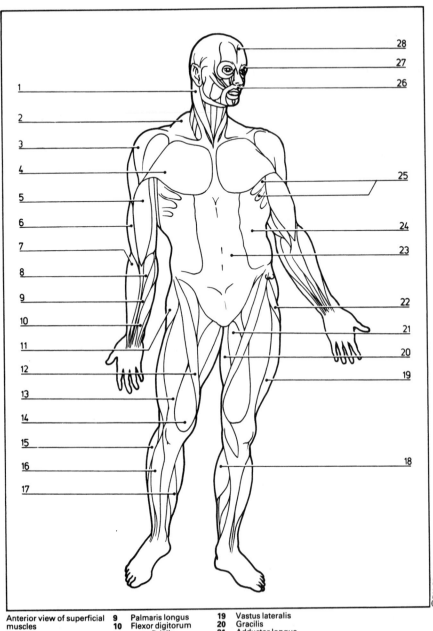

Anterior view of superficial muscles

1	Sternocleidomastoid	**9**	Palmaris longus	**19**	Vastus lateralis
2	Trapezius	**10**	Flexor digitorum superficialis	**20**	Gracilis
3	Deltoid	**11**	Gluteus medius	**21**	Adductor longus
4	Pectoralis major	**12**	Sartorius	**22**	Tensor fasciae latae
5	Biceps brachii	**13**	Rectus femoris	**23**	Rectus abdominis
6	Brachialis	**14**	Vastus medialis	**24**	External abdominal oblique
7	Brachioradialis	**15**	Peroneus longus	**25**	Serratus anterior
8	Flexor carpi radialis	**16**	Tibialis anterior	**26**	Orbicularis oris
		17	Soleus	**27**	Orbicularis oculi
		18	Gastrocnemius	**28**	Occipitofrontalis

16   THE NEW W.E.T. WORKOUT

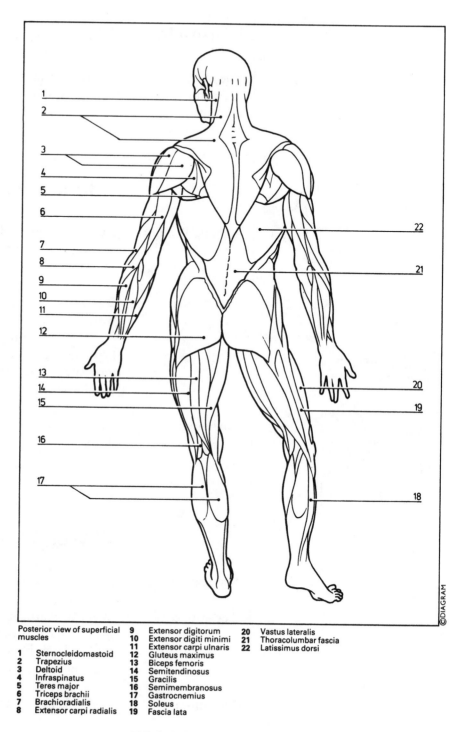

Posterior view of superficial muscles

1 Sternocleidomastoid
2 Trapezius
3 Deltoid
4 Infraspinatus
5 Teres major
6 Triceps brachii
7 Brachioradialis
8 Extensor carpi radialis
9 Extensor digitorum
10 Extensor digiti minimi
11 Extensor carpi ulnaris
12 Gluteus maximus
13 Biceps femoris
14 Semitendinosus
15 Gracilis
16 Semimembranosus
17 Gastrocnemius
18 Soleus
19 Fascia lata
20 Vastus lateralis
21 Thoracolumbar fascia
22 Latissimus dorsi

©DIAGRAM

Warm-Up/Cool-Down W.E.T.s

The following are suggested warm-up and cool-down exercises, each illustrated and with its starting position and technique described.

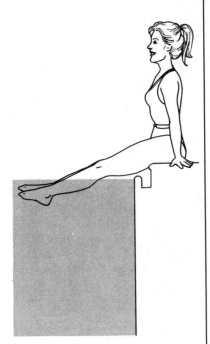

TOE TESTER

Starting Position: Sit on the edge of the pool with your legs in the water. Put your hands on your hips for support.

Technique: Begin with foot circles: move your feet inward, downward, outward, and upward in a circular motion. With your knees slightly bent, use an alternative up-and-down leg movement (flutter kick), keeping your ankles loose.

Variation: Try a breaststroke or frog kick and some leg crossovers.

WATER WALKING

Starting Position: Stand in chest-deep water.

Technique: Walk forward, moving through the water, using hands in opposition, e.g., right foot forward, left hand forward. Use the edge of the pool for support, if needed.

Variation: Walk backward and sideward.

TRICEPS STRETCH

Starting Position: Stand in waist- to chin-deep water, feet hip-width apart.

Technique: Extend your left arm over your head, palm facing in. Grasp your left elbow with your right hand, bending it and guiding the left arm to reach behind your head, resting your hand at the base of your neck. Gently pull on the left elbow for additional stretch. Release and reverse arms.

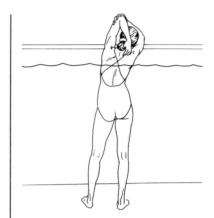

CROSS CHEST STRETCH

Starting Position: Stand in chin- to chest-deep water, feet shoulder-width apart.

Technique: Extend your right arm in front of your body, with thumb pointing up. With your left hand, grasp your right arm underneath the elbow and hold right arm close to your chest under your chin. Repeat with the other arm.

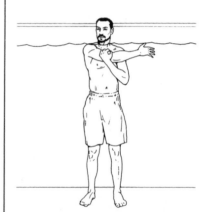

STANDING TALL

Starting Position: Standing in shoulder-deep water, place your back against the pool wall.

Technique: Press your back, head, shoulders, buttocks, and heels against the wall. Take one step away from the wall, keeping your back straight in line with your head. Return to the wall by taking a step backward and rechecking your position.

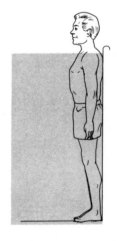

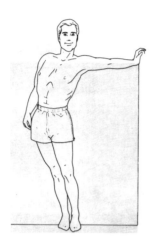

ARM STRETCH

Starting Position: In chest-deep water stand arms distance from wall with inside hand on the wall for support.

Technique: Slowly stretch upper body by pressing one shoulder forward and hold for 30 seconds. Change arms and repeat.

AQUA LUNGE

Starting Position: Face the pool wall and hold the edge with both hands, shoulder-width apart. Place your feet against the wall in a straddle position, beyond shoulder-width.

Technique: Shift your body weight to the right, bending the right knee, while the left leg is extended. Hold the stretch. Return to center and shift your body weight to the left.

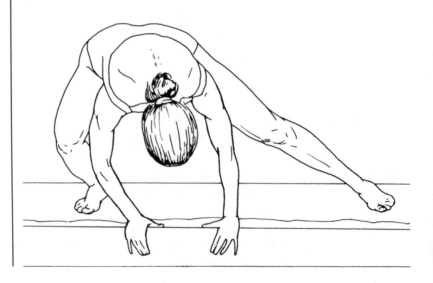

PIKE BODY STRETCH

Starting Position: Facing the wall, hold onto the pool edge with both your hands; bend your knees and place your toes against the wall below your hands.

Technique: Slowly extend your legs and arms into a piked position and hold it. Place your heels flat against the wall. Gradually return to starting position.

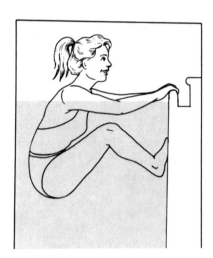 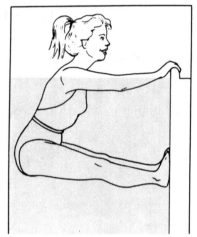

LEG SPLIT

Starting Position: Stand facing the pool wall in waist-deep water, both hands on the edge; turn out your feet and place them where the wall and bottom meet.

Technique: Move legs outward towards a split position by alternately placing feet beyond hip width.

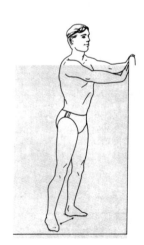

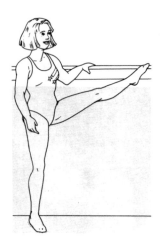

BALLET LEG STRETCH

Starting Position: Standing in waist-deep water parallel to the pool wall, place one foot on the edge.

Technique: Grasp the wall with one hand and slowly straighten your knee, lowering your body as close to your leg as possible. Hold for 30 seconds. Change legs and repeat.

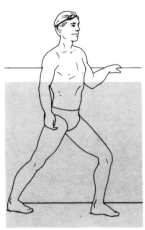

RUNNER'S CALF STRETCH

Starting Position: Stand in chest-deep water, facing the pool wall.

Technique: Move your right leg behind body backward and stretch the calf muscle by pressing your heel to the pool's bottom. Repeat with the other foot. Change to other side.

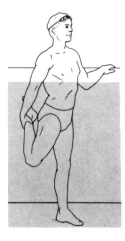

RUNNER'S QUADRICEPS STRETCH

Starting Position: Stand in chest-deep water. Grasp the deck with your left hand for support.

Technique: Bend your right leg behind you, with heel toward the buttock. Grasping your right foot with your right hand, pull your foot upward, stretching thigh muscle (quadriceps), while keeping knees close together. Hold for a count of five. Lower your foot and repeat with the left leg.

HEAD CIRCLES

Starting Position: Stand in neck-deep water, your hands at your sides.

Technique: Slowly rotate your head in a clockwise, then counterclockwise, motion. Lift your head forward; then lower it backward.

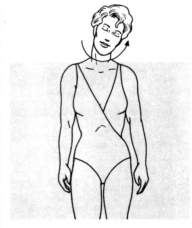

SHOULDER SHRUG

Starting Position: Stand in shoulder-deep water, your arms at your sides.

Technique: Lift your shoulders up and down together; then alternate left and right shoulder shrugs. Bring both shoulders forward, then backward.

Variation: Try "chicken wings." Place your hands on your shoulders and rotate your arms and shoulders in a circle.

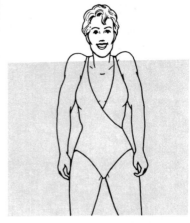

OVERHEAD STRETCH

Starting Position: With both hands, grasp either end of a wand, stick, or rolled-up towel. Place it behind your neck.

Technique: Either in water or on land, extend your arms over your head. Stretch your body by moving your arms gradually from left to right, keeping your arms straight.

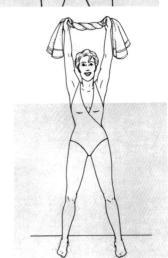

Main W.E.T.s

Upper Body W.E.T.s

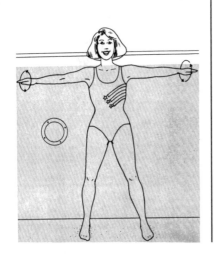

For each W.E.T., I've provided a description of the starting position and of the technique; in addition, there are illustrations. I've also given you a choice between a relaxed and a vigorous or energetic variation of each W.E.T. Depending on your needs, energy, time, and ability, you can choose the appropriate variation. It helps to establish the standard technique before trying a variation.

These upper, middle, and lower-body W.E.T.s can be combined to help you improve your coordination and utilize more muscle groups.

ARM AND WRIST SWIRLS

Starting Position: Stand in shoulder-deep water. Extend your arms out from your sides and submerge them, bending your knees slightly.

Technique: Keeping your arms straight, rotate them in forward circles. Then reverse to backward circles. Flex your wrists up and down as you rotate your arms.

Variation:

Relaxed: Create smaller, slower circles.

Energetic: Create larger, more vigorous circles, using hand paddles for added resistance.

SPORT SWINGS (AND FOLLOW-THROUGH)

Starting Position: Stand in chest-deep water, your arms out at your sides.

Technique: Move one arm forward, as if you were swinging a racquet. Follow through and recover out of the water; then swing your arm backward into the starting position. Repeat with the other arm.

Variation:

Relaxed: Practice a half swing, stopping before you follow through. Keep your swing arm on the surface of the water to decrease resistance.

W.E.T. TIP

Especially beneficial for tennis, paddle tennis, badminton, racquetball, squash, golf, baseball, bowling, and fencing; helps improve overhand swings, backhand swings, forehand swings, and underhand swings.

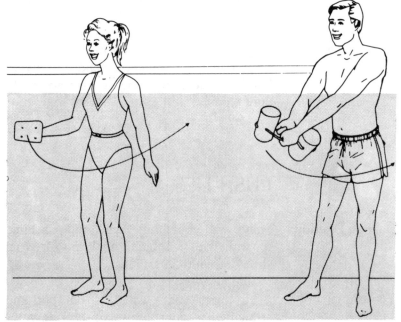

Tennis Swing

Golf Swing

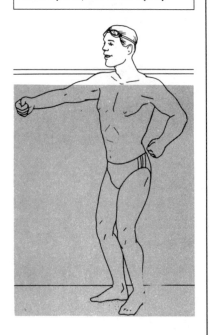

SPORT ARM PUMP

Starting Position: Stand in chest-deep water with your feet shoulder-width apart.

Technique: With your fists closed, alternate your arms in a vigorous punching motion at shoulder level in front of you.

Variation:

Relaxed: Move your arms with a slower, longer follow-through, straightening your elbows fully on each arm extension.

Energetic: Pump your arms more vigorously to create greater water turbulence; make the water "boil" by just breaking the surface with your elbows.

PUSH-UPS

Starting Position: Stand with your body facing and touching the wall, with your hands on the pool's edge, shoulder-width apart.

Technique: Bend knees and push off from bottom, straightening your elbows and lifting your upper body out of the water.

Variation:

Relaxed: Stand at arms' distance from the side of the pool with your elbows locked. Bring your chest to the pool edge by bending your elbows.

Energetic: Hold the push-up position for three or more seconds.

Try the push-up in water too deep for your feet to touch bottom.

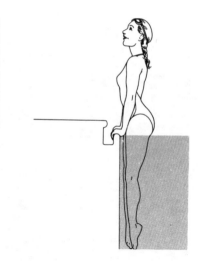

SCULL AND HUG

Starting Position: Stand in chin-deep water, your arms extended in front of you with the thumbs pointing downward.

Technique: Sweep your arms out and back as far as possible, pressing the water backward and keeping your thumbs down. Then turn your thumbs up and press the water forward, until your arms hug your body.

Variation:

Relaxed: Turn your hands so that the palms face the pool bottom as you sweep your arms outward and forward. Bend your elbows as you sweep your arms.

Energetic: Use hand paddles for extra resistance, and to gain added flexibility try to touch your hands behind your back.

W.E.T. TIP

This is great practice for your sculling motion used in treading.

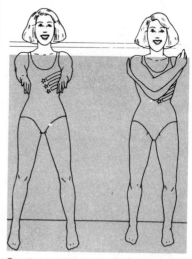

Starting position   Ending position

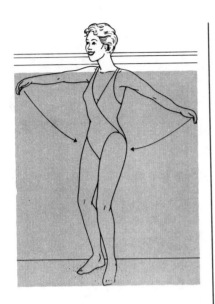

WATER PUSH

Starting Position: Stand in chest-deep water, your right arm extended behind you and your left arm stretched out in front of you.

Technique: With palms facing down, press both arms toward the pool's bottom, then upward toward the surface in an underwater semicircle. Hold and repeat.

Variation:

Relaxed: Move your hand through a shorter range.

Energetic: Exercise with hand paddles in chin-deep water.

HANG "10"

Starting Position: Stand with your back against the pool wall. Reach over your shoulders and grasp the pool edge with your hands more than shoulder-width apart.

Technique: Bend your knees so that your feet lift off the pool bottom, allowing the weight of your body to stretch your arms and upper body, with the water's buoyancy supporting your lower body.

Relax your head and neck muscles and breathe deeply as you stretch. Hold stretch for 5 to 10 seconds.

Variation:

Relaxed: Use the corner of the pool for greater comfort and support.

Energetic:	To increase the stretch, move your hands closer together.

REAR PUSH-UPS

Starting Position:	Stand in waist-deep water with your back against the wall. Place your hands on the pool edge close to your sides, with your fingers pointing toward the water.
Technique:	Bend knees and jump up, straightening your elbows and lifting your upper body out of the water. For those with limited upper body strength, begin with the relaxed variation.
Variation:	
Relaxed:	Begin in the corner of the pool for greater leverage.
Energetic:	Hold the push-up position for three or more seconds. Bring your legs into an L or piked position after you lift.

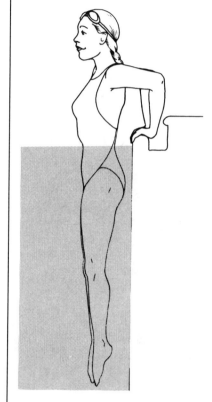

MEDLEY OF STROKES

Starting Position:	Stand in shoulder-deep water.
Technique:	Keeping your feet on the pool bottom, use the crawl stroke, breaststroke, butterfly, backstroke, or the sidestroke arm motion.
Variation:	
Relaxed:	Stand in waist-deep water while practicing whatever stroke or strokes you wish.

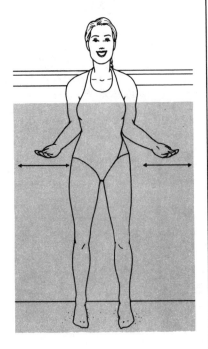

Energetic: Combine all the strokes into a medley of strokes.

Consult chapter 6, W.E.T. Drills to Swim Skills, for an extensive look at all of the strokes mentioned above.

SCULLING

Starting Position: Stand in shoulder-deep water with your feet almost together, knees bent. Extend your arms behind your hips under the surface and close to each other.

Technique: Move your hands in a figure-eight motion: turn your palms downward and outward and press your hands out past shoulder-width, keeping your upper arms relatively motionless.

Then turn your palms inward and press your hands in until they almost touch.

Then turn your palms outward and repeat the movement.

Variation:

Relaxed: Stand in shoulder-deep water, knees bent, with your arms extended forward under the surface of the water. Practice figure-eight sculling arm motion, arms extending out to shoulder level.

Energetic: Keep sculling motion under hips from a back-float position with a continuous upward scull.

See chapter 9, Synchronized Swimming, for additional sculling W.E.T.s.

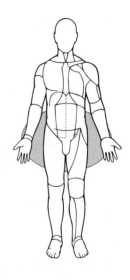

SIT-UPS

Starting Position: Float on your back, your hands holding the pool's edge.

Technique: Bend your knees and bring them toward your chest. Then extend your legs again.

Variation:

Relaxed: Use the corner of the pool for extra leverage.

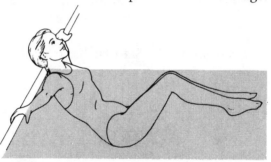

Energetic: For a very vigorous sit-up, float on your back, your knees bent and your calves resting on the pool deck. Supporting your head with your hands, tuck your chin up to your chest, then lie back into the starting position.

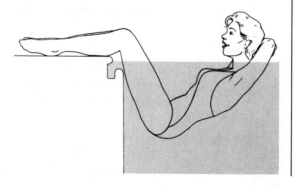

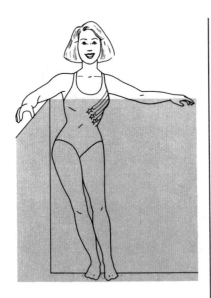

HIP TOUCH

Starting Position: Stand in chest-deep water, perpendicular to the pool wall and one arm's length from it.

Technique: Keeping your feet on the bottom, touch your hip to the wall, then pull your hip as far away from the wall as possible. Repeat on the other side.

Variation:

Relaxed: Stand closer to the wall. Shift your weight from one foot to the other, rocking your hips from side to side.

Energetic: Start farther from the wall.

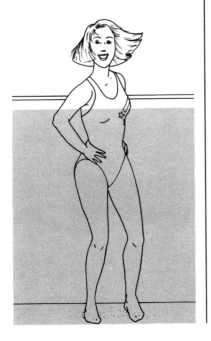

TRUNK TWIST

Starting Position: Stand in chest-deep water with hands on your hips.

Technique: Inhale as you twist your body to one side, then exhale as you return to the starting position. Repeat on the opposite side.

Variation:

Relaxed: Twist only your shoulders and head to each side without coordinating breathing.

Energetic: Extend your arms out from your sides underwater, keeping them parallel to the water's surface throughout the exercise.

OVERHEAD SWAY

Starting Position: Stand in waist-deep water with your feet shoulder-width apart. Extend your arms overhead.

Technique: Sway your arms overhead from side to side, feeling the reach in your rib cage.

Variation:

Relaxed: Sway with your hands behind your head.

Energetic: Keeping your arms together, sway them in a counterclockwise circle across the front of your body, over the surface of the water and back to an overhead position. Change directions.

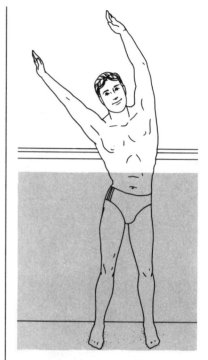

CIRCLE SPRAY

Starting Position: Stand in waist-deep water with your arms extended to your sides and your fingers at the water's surface. Stand with feet shoulder-width apart for balance, knees and hips slightly flexed.

Technique: Turn slowly in one direction as far as you can, keeping your feet stationary and your arms straight. Your fingertips should spray the water as you move. Breathe normally.

Turn your torso slowly back until you are facing front; then turn as far as you can in the opposite direction.

Slowly return again to the center position. Letting the heel of your trailing leg lift and turn will allow full range of motion.

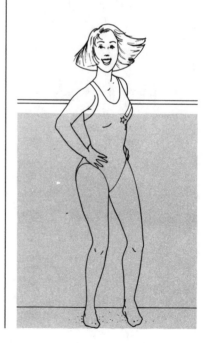

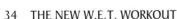

Variation:

Relaxed: Keep fingers higher on water's surface.

Energetic: Keep your fingers lower in the water.

BUTTOCK SQUEEZE

Starting Position: Stand with your back in a corner of the pool, one hand on either edge and your elbows bent.

Technique: Press your hips forward and tighten your buttocks. Then relax your buttocks and allow your hips to return close to the wall, and repeat.

Variation:

Relaxed: Squeeze your buttocks together without pressing your hips forward.

Energetic: Add a pelvic tilt to the buttock squeeze and bring your body to a back float position.

KNEE TUCK

Starting Position: Stand in chest-deep water, with your back against the wall.

Technique: Grasp one knee and bring it toward your chest. Then release your leg and extend it forward by straightening the leg. Return the leg to the starting position.

Starting position

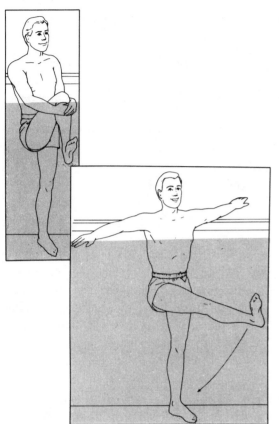

Variation:

Relaxed: Hold onto the pool edge for support. Bend the knee and bring the leg up without grasping the knee. Return the leg to the starting position.

Energetic: Pull your knee toward your chest as high as possible, then straighten your leg from the knee close to the water's surface before returning to the starting position.

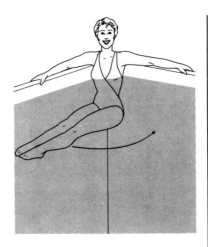

CORNER LEG SWING

Starting Position: Stand with your back to the corner of the pool in any depth of water, one hand on either edge and with your arms slightly bent.

Technique: Pike at the waist by lifting your legs, creating an L with your body. Maintain the L as you twist your body and swing your legs first to the right, then to the left.

Variation:

Relaxed: Bend your knees as you swing your legs.

Energetic: Extend your arms for a wider starting position. Lift your body in an L shape and swing your legs from right to left, touching your toes to each wall.

BODY WAVE

Starting Position: Stand close to the wall in chin-deep water, holding onto the wall with one hand.

Technique: With legs together, press your hips alternately forward and backward, keeping your knees relaxed and allowing your hips and legs to perform a sinuous, wavelike motion.

Variation:

Relaxed: Face the wall, holding on with both hands.

Energetic: Begin in deep water, holding the wall for support, and use a vigorous dolphin leg motion to move your body in a wavelike motion.

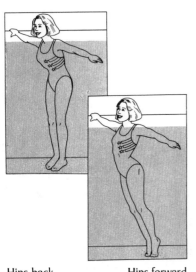

Hips back   Hips forward

BACK EXTENSION

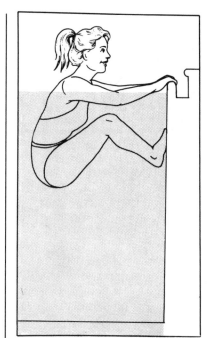

Starting Position: Facing wall, hold onto the pool wall with arms shoulder-width apart in bracket position, and place feet on the wall slightly farther apart than arms. Place the ball of each foot on the wall.

Technique: Slowly extend your legs behind you into a streamlined prone float position. Inhale. Use your abdominal muscles to lift and control your legs until your feet are at the water's surface and separated slightly.

Bend your knees toward your chest. Exhale. Using your abdominal muscles to bring your feet to the wall, return to your starting position.

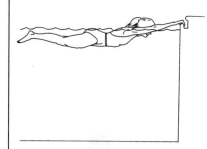

Variation:

Relaxed: Place your hands in a bracket position for better support. (Grasp the pool edge with one hand and place the other hand flat against the pool wall with fingertips pointed down.)

Energetic: For a more energetic exercise, place feet in a flotation device to increase the effort needed to bring your feet to the wall, helping to strengthen your abdominal muscles. Control your legs as they return to the water's surface, being careful not to arch your back.

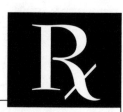

If you have back problems, ask your doctor's advice before doing this exercise.

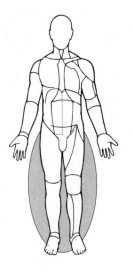

LEG SWIRL

Starting Position: Stand perpendicular to the pool wall, grasping the pool edge with your inside hand.

Technique: Lift your outside leg in front of you as comfortably high as you can. Then slowly swing your leg around in a half circle until your leg is extended just behind your. Breathe regularly.

Slowly swing your leg back to the front and lower it.

Turn around and swing the other leg. Do the same number of repetitions on each side, beginning with a comfortable number and progressing.

Variation:

Relaxed: Foot Circles: Stand perpendicular to the pool wall, grasping the pool edge with your inside hand. Lift your outside leg in front of you and trace a small circle in the water with your foot in a clockwise direction. Follow this by tracing a circle in a counterclockwise direction. Do the same number of repetitions of each movement for each leg.

Energetic: Try to bring your leg as close to the surface of the water as you swirl your leg around, keeping your posture erect, creating a larger circle.

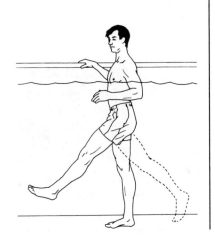

AQUA-JOG

Starting Position: Begin in chest-deep water.

Technique: Run in place or alternate directions (forward, backward, sideways, diagonally, in circles, etc.).

Variation:

Relaxed: Skip in place. Perform the exercise in shallow water.

Energetic: Move in several directions—forward, backward, sideways—taking longer strides. Run in deeper water.

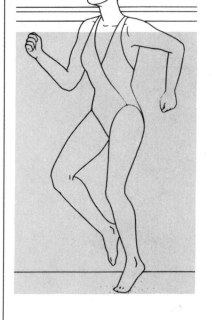

ROCKETTE KICK

Starting Position: Stand in chest-deep water, your back against the pool wall. Hold onto the pool edge for support.

Technique: Lift one leg at a time to the water's surface, keeping your knees locked.

Variation:

Relaxed: Bend your knee as you lift your leg.

Energetic: Use a pull-buoy under your heel for extra resistance. Flex your foot to keep the buoy in place. Bring your leg as high as possible, and keep your knees straight.

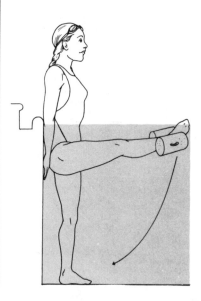

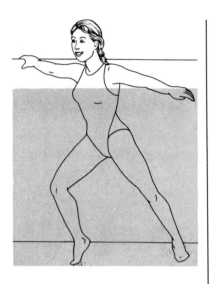

LEG LUNGE

Starting Position: Stand in waist-deep water.

Technique: Take one large lunge-step forward with your right foot, the right knee bent and the left leg straight. Press the body weight through your hips to feel the stretch on the inner thigh. This exercise can also be done by stepping sideways (as in a fencing lunge) as far as possible. Return to a standing position and repeat on the other side.

Variation:

Relaxed: Use a smaller lunge step.

Energetic: Stand in chest-deep water. Jump to change leg positions, keeping your weight on the forward leg. Hold each lunge position longer for an extra stretch.

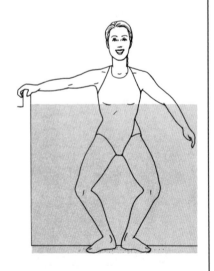

PLIÉ SQUEEZE

Starting Position: Stand in waist-deep water, holding onto the edge of the pool for balance. Touch your heels together and turn your toes outward.

Technique: Make a deep-knee bend (plié), then squeeze your buttocks together as you straighten up. Keep your hips in line with your shoulders throughout.

Variation:

Relaxed: Squeeze your buttocks, bending your knees only slightly.

Energetic:	Repeat the plié squeeze with your feet shoulder-width apart. (Ballet lovers: do the plié in all six ballet positions.)	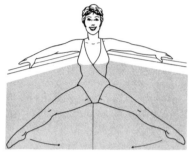

LEG CROSSOVER

Starting Position:	Put your arms over the sides of the pool and place your back against the wall. Lift your legs to a 90° angle, keeping them straight and together.

Leg crossover, starting position

Technique:	Separate your legs into a V; then bring them back together. Alternately open and close your legs. Maintain the L shape, and keep your legs straight.

Variation:

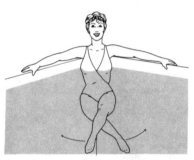

Relaxed:	Bend your knee to form a 90° angle, and place one leg over the other, knees crossed in a sitting position.

Leg crossover, middle position. Next return legs to starting position.

Energetic:	Begin by opening your legs as far as possible. Keeping your left leg stationary, bring the right completely over to meet the left one; then return to open position. Repeat with the other leg.

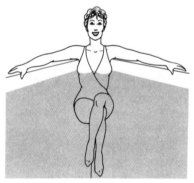

AQUA DANCER

Starting Position:	Stand in chest-deep water, your feet together.

Leg crossover, relaxed position

Technique:	Bend your knees and move your body from side to side in a step-together-step dance sequence.

Relaxed: Try the slower dance steps, e.g., fox-trot, waltz, etc.

Energetic: Try the more vigorous dance steps, e.g., square dances. Point and flex your feet in square-dance style (bringing your elbows up just under your chest).

SIDE SWIPE

Starting Position: Rest your arms and hands lightly on the deck and stand with your back against the wall at the corner.

Technique: Alternately bring one leg out to the side, then down and across your standing leg toward the opposite wall in a semicircular pattern.

Variation:

Relaxed: Move your leg in a smaller circle, bending the knee if necessary.

Energetic: For extra resistance, place your heel between the floats of a pull-buoy. Try the exercise without holding onto the wall.

WALL WALK

Starting Position: Stand in the pool at a comfortable depth, facing the pool wall. Grasp the pool edge with both hands.

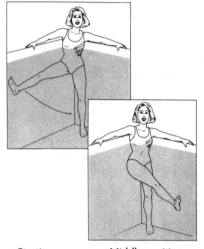

Starting position.

Middle position. Next return leg to starting position.

Technique:	Place your feet flat on the pool wall just above the pool floor.
	Slowly walk up the wall, no farther than waist level, breathing normally.
	Then return to a standing position by slowly walking down the pool wall.

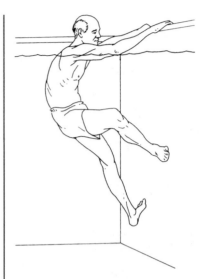

Variation:

Relaxed:	Hold onto the pool edge with both feet flat on the pool wall just above the pool bottom. With feet shoulder-width apart, bend and flex your legs.
Energetic:	Walk with bigger steps alternately to the right and to the left.

LEG TREADING

Starting Position:	Begin in chin-deep water, one hand resting lightly on the pool edge, a safety line, or a buoy.
Technique:	Use one or more of the following leg motions: ❑ frog kick (knees apart) ❑ whip kick (knees close together) ❑ bicycle leg motion ❑ scissor kick (as in sidestroke)

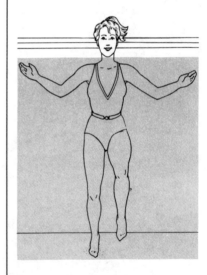

Variation:

Relaxed:	Using a flotation device (e.g., kickboard, pull-buoy, arm float) to support your upper body while you practice leg treading.
Energetic:	Keep your hands as high out of the water as possible while treading. (This leg tread is used by water-polo players and synchronized swimmers.)

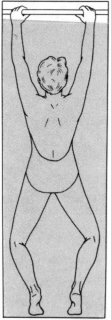
Breaststroke kick

MEDLEY OF KICKS

Starting Position: Face the pool wall and assume the bracket position, i.e., hold onto the edge with one hand and press the other hand against the wall under the water, fingers pointing downward. Then pull with the top hand and press with the bottom hand as you lift your legs to the surface.

Variation:

Relaxed: Pick one leg motion and kick gently.

Energetic: Combine all the above kicks into a medley. Kick vigorously.

Consult chapter 6, W.E.T. Drills to Swim Skills, for instructions on combining these kicks with the proper upper-body movements.

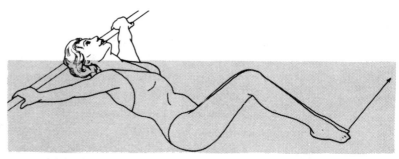
Supine dolphin kick

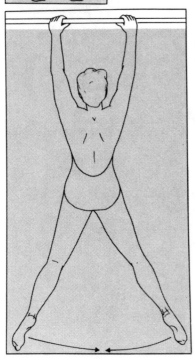

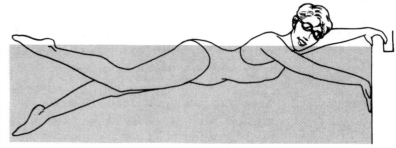
Flutter kick

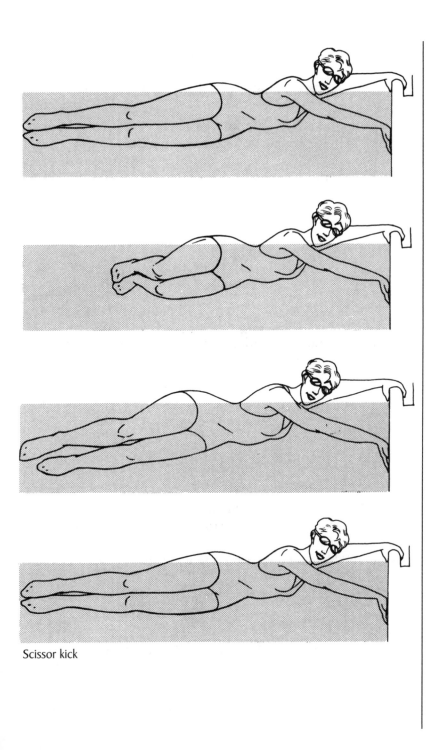

Scissor kick

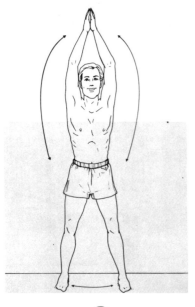

The following are sample total body W.E.T.s that combine various muscle groups, which will be presented and highlighted throughout the W.E.T. Workout program.

Some of the preceding W.E.T.s have been combined to provide combination W.E.T.s. Create your own as you become more familiar with the program.

AQUA JUMPING JACKS

Begin by standing in deep water. Turn your palms upward and touch them overhead as you separate your legs into a V position. Return to the starting position by turning your palms downward and bringing them back to your sides as you bring your legs together.

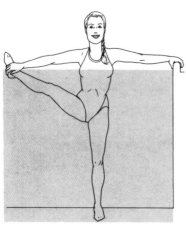

BALLET V

An arm and leg stretch-out. Standing in chest-deep water, grasp your right inside heel with your right hand and slowly straighten your knees while balancing on your left. Return to starting position by bending both arms and legs simultaneously.

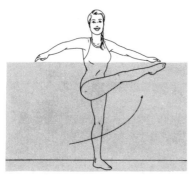

CROSSOVER TOE TOUCH

Standing in chest-deep water, lift your right leg and tap your left hand to your right foot. Alternate with your right hand touching your left foot.

COORDINATED SPORT ARM
AND LEG MOTIONS

Practice your favorite sport motion, coordinating arm and leg action. See chapter 5, Sport Cross-training W.E.T.s, for examples.

Coordinate the arm motions of the following strokes in chest-deep water.

The Freestyler   Begin in chest-deep water for all strokes. As you do an aqua jog, use the crawl-stroke arm motion; add rhythmic breathing by turning your head to one side as your opposite arm is extended.

The Backstroker   As you aqua jog backward, use backstroke arm motion.

The Breaststroker   With forward aqua jog or jump use a breast-stroke arm motion. Keep arms underwater for the outward scull motion and recovery. Add your breathing by lifting head at the start of your pull.

The Sidestroker   With a sideways aqua jog, pull and press arms using a sidestroke arm motion.

The Butterflyer   With forward aqua-jog, use butterfly arm motion. Create large forward arm circles with both arms, hands simultaneously pulling through the water.

PENDULUM BODY SWING

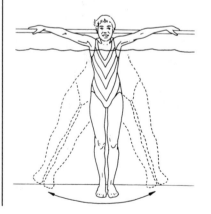

Stand with legs together in neck-deep water with your back against the pool wall. Grasp the pool with both hands. Pull with your right arm and push with your left arm to swing your legs sideways and upward toward your right arm. Then return to a vertical position. Repeat in the other direction. Inhale through your nose as you swing your legs up, and exhale through your mouth as you lower them.

TREADING

In treading, you use the arms and legs to maintain a vertical position in deep water with little energy. Begin in a sitting position, with your shoulders over your knees, in chin-deep water. The arms perform a wide sculling motion, while the legs can use any of the following motions: a bicycle leg motion, scissor kick, frog kick, whip kick, or eggbeater motion.

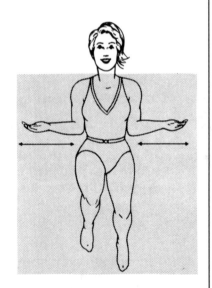

TUG-OF-WAR

In chin-deep water, use a reverse scull as you tread with your legs. The scull will press you underwater while the treading will keep you up. See which is *your* better half!

CREATE YOUR OWN STROKE

Combine different leg motions with different arm motions, for example, from a back float position, use backward arm circles (butterfly arms) with a frog kick (breaststroke leg motion).

Progressive 12-Week W.E.T. Workout Program

3

Now you're ready to take the plunge to begin your progressive 12-week program. Why 12 weeks? Because three months (a season's training) is a realistic period of time for getting into shape. In these 12 weeks you'll be able to develop a weekly routine of doing W.E.T.s. I recommend that you do your W.E.T.s three times per week (every other day is best). However, if your schedule won't accommodate this, do the best you can. (You'll benefit from doing your W.E.T.s even once a week!)

The following chart outlines your level of fitness from week 1 to week 12 and beyond.

W.E.T. Workout Components

All the suggested W.E.T.s (*Water Exercise Techniques*) that make up each workout are described in the preceding W.E.T. section. Each W.E.T. workout contains the following components:

SHAKE OUT

As part of you W.E.T. set, do a "shake out" between segments for each body part. The shake out is a rest period to help reenergize, loosen, and relax your muscles before you begin the next part of the W.E.T. set. Think of the shake out as a shimmy. Bob up and down, relax, and shake your arms and legs. Take up to a minute for each "shake out." The "shake out" helps get rid of excess lactic acid. The main energy fuel the body uses is simple sugar (glucose), which is broken down into carbon dioxide and water by a series of complex steps. In the absence of sufficient oxygen, the breakdown process is incomplete and larger than normal amounts of lactic acid tend to accumulate in the blood.

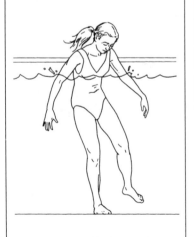

Warm-Up

As I've already noted, the warm-up is an important part of your workout. *Don't skip it!* It gets you moving, it gets the blood flowing, and it prepares your body for the W.E.T. set. It also prepares your joints and muscles to move more easily through their full range of motion. Your warm-up should also include a comfortable adjustment to the water (water walking is a great technique for this).

Main W.E.T. Set

This is the "meat and potatoes" portion of your workout. Each main set includes W.E.T.s for each body area—upper, middle, lower—as well as exercises to improve your coordination. As you become more fit, your W.E.T. set will increase in duration from 10 minutes to 20 minutes or more. Arrange the exercises as you desire, but be sure you do the exercises for each body part. To help you remember your main W.E.T. set, jot it down on a 3 x 5 card and place it at poolside. In each W.E.T. set, there are optional relaxed and energetic segments. Let your preference, energy, time, and ability dictate how you will exercise. As you progress, challenge yourself with the more energetic variations.

Cool-Down

The cool-down segment of your workout helps your body to slow down and relax, gradually bringing your heart rate and breathing back to your normal resting rate. The stretch-out should last about five minutes.

How to Improve Your F.I.T.ness with Your 12-Week Progressive W.E.T. Workout Program

1st Month (Weeks 1–4)

Welcome to the 12-Week Progressive Workout Program. If you are just starting to get in condition, these first weeks are an ideal "bridge" to a lifetime of fun and fitness. If the W.E.T. Workout® program is an addition to your ongoing fitness program, whether as an alternate activity, cross-training or for therapeutic purposes, use these first four weeks to explore the benefits of water for your conditioning goals.

In the first month, your main W.E.T. set should last approximately 10 minutes. Each exercise is performed for approximately 1 minute or a specific number of repetitions. Remember your 5-minute warm-up and 5-minute cool-down, for a total 20-minute water workout.

2nd Month (Weeks 5–8)

Enjoy your program! Your main W.E.T. set increases by 5 minutes and is now approximately 15 minutes in length. Try the optional swim equipment, and check your pulse.

3rd Month (Weeks 9–12)

You're on your way to using Water Exercise Techniques for aerobic fitness. Your main W.E.T. set increases by 5 minutes, becoming 20 minutes in length. Try new workout variations.

Weeks 13 and Beyond

Maintain your new level of F.I.T.ness. You can have more fun by varying your W.E.T. workouts.
    Many other W.E.T.s are described throughout this book.
    Creatively combine various W.E.T.s to suit your interests.

Other W.E.T. Workout® variations are described in the following section. These include water activities in spas, family and partner members, open-water, and more.

F.I.T. PRINCIPLE

As you become more F.I.T., try:

Frequency	❑ Increasing the number of workouts per week.
	❑ Increasing the number of repetitions per exercise.
	❑ Increasing the number of W.E.T.s per workout.
Intensity	❑ Increasing the intensity of your W.E.T.s with fins, hand paddles, etc.
	❑ Increasing the difficulty of your W.E.T.s from relaxed to energetic.
Time	❑ Increasing the length of your main set up to 40 minutes
	❑ Increasing or varying the length of time devoted to each W.E.T.

12-Week Progressive Workout

WEEK 1

You've taken the plunge and are off to a great start. Try to do your W.E.T. workout every other day.

Comments:
F.I.T. (e.g., THR, time, number of reps)

WARM-UP (5 min.)	**Toe Tester** **Water Walking** **Standing Tall**		_____ _____ _____
W.E.T. SET (10 min.) approx. 1 minute per exercise	**Upper:**	**Water Push** **Push-Ups—** **Relaxed**	_____ _____
	Shake Out		
	Middle:	**Trunk Twist** **Sit-Ups**	_____ _____
	Shake Out		
	Lower:	**Leg Swirl** **Side Swipe**	_____ _____
	Shake Out		
	Combination: The Freestyler		_____
COOL-DOWN (5 min.)	**Arm Stretch** **Aqua Lunge** **Runner's Quadriceps Stretch**		_____ _____ _____

WEEK 2

You may be experiencing some muscle soreness. Don't worry; your body will become adjusted to your W.E.T. program. Stay with it!

Comments:

WARM-UP (5 min.)	**Overhead Stretch** **Water Walking** **Leg Split**		_____ _____ _____
W.E.T. SET (10 min.)	**Upper:**	**Arm and Wrist Swirls** **Rear Push-Ups**	_____ _____
	Shake Out		
	Middle:	**Body Wave** **Back Extension**	_____ _____
	Shake Out		
	Lower:	**Medley of Kicks** **Leg Lunge**	_____ _____
	Shake Out		
	Combination:	**Treading**	_____
COOL-DOWN (5 min.)	**Shoulder Shrug** **Cross Chest Stretch** **Ballet Leg Stretch**		_____ _____ _____

WEEK 3

Use the W.E.T. sport skills you like and know for the combination.

Comments:

WARM-UP   **Water Walking**   _____
(5 min.)   **Head Circles**   _____
    Triceps Stretch   _____

W.E.T. SET   **Upper:**   **Scull and Hug**   _____
(10 min.)   **Sport Swings**   _____

Shake Out

    Middle: **Circle Spray**   _____
    Overhead Sway   _____

Shake Out

    Lower: **Leg Crossover**   _____
    Aqua-Jog   _____

Shake Out

    Combination: **Coordinated Sport**
    Arm and
    Leg Motions
    Ballet V   _____

COOL-DOWN   **Runner's Quadriceps Stretch**   _____
(5 min.)   **Shoulder Shrug**   _____
    Head Circles   _____

WEEK 4

Inner fitness: What you see is not all you get! Your W.E.T. workouts are designed to improve your aerobic capacity too!

Comments:

WARM-UP (5 min.)	**Toe Tester** **Runner's Calf Stretch** **Cross Chest Stretch**		_____ _____ _____
W.E.T. SET (10 min.)	**Upper:**	**Medley of Strokes** **Water Push**	_____ _____
	Shake Out		
	Middle:	**Hip Touch** **Circle Spray**	_____ _____
	Shake Out		
	Lower:	**Leg Crossover** **Plié Squeeze**	_____ _____
	Shake Out		
	Combination:	**The Breaststroker** **Crossover Toe Touch**	_____ _____
COOL-DOWN (5 min.)	**Water Walking** **Aqua Lunge** **Standing Tall**		_____ _____ _____

WEEK 5

Congratulations! After 4 weeks, you're getting into shape with your W.E.T. workouts. Your bonus is five minutes added to your main set. You're ready!

Comments:

WARM-UP (5 min.)	**Water Walking** **Pike Body Stretch** **Shoulder Shrug**		_____ _____ _____
W.E.T. SET (15 min.— add 5 minutes)	**Upper:**	**Push-Ups** **Sculling** **Sport Arm Pump**	_____ _____ _____
	Shake Out		
	Middle:	**Sit-Ups** **Back Extension** **Trunk Twist**	_____ _____ _____
	Shake Out		
	Lower:	**Rockette Kick** **Leg Swirl** **Aqua-Jog**	_____ _____ _____
	Shake Out		
	Combination: The Backstroker **Tug-of-War**		_____ _____
COOL-DOWN (5 min.)	**Runner's Calf Stretch** **Arm Stretch** **Overhead Stretch**		_____ _____ _____

WEEK 6

Use aquatic exercise equipment for variety: e.g., fins (for legs), or hand paddles (for arms), etc.

Comments:

WARM-UP (5 min.)	**Toe Tester** **Aqua Lunge** **Leg Split**		_____ _____ _____
W.E.T. SET (15 min.)	**Upper:**	**Scull and Hug** **Water Push** **Medley of Strokes**	_____ _____ _____
	Shake Out		
	Middle:	**Buttock Squeeze** **Circle Spray** **Body Wave**	_____ _____ _____
	Shake Out		
	Lower:	**Side Swipe** **Medley of Kicks** **Wall Walk**	_____ _____ _____
	Shake Out		
	Combination:	**Aqua Jumping Jacks** **The Freestyler**	_____ _____
COOL-DOWN (5 min.)	**Arm Stretch** **Ballet Leg Stretch** **Runner's Quadriceps Stretch**		_____ _____ _____

WEEK 7

Try some new upper-body techniques and the Butterflyer. Remember to check your pulse.

Comments:

WARM-UP (5 min.)	Water Walking Shoulder Shrug Pike Body Stretch		_____ _____ _____
W.E.T. SET (15 min.)	**Upper:**	Hang "10" Arm and Wrist Swirls Sculling	_____ _____ _____
	Shake Out		
	Middle:	Hip Touch Corner Leg Swing Knee Tuck	_____ _____ _____
	Shake Out/Pulse Check		
	Lower:	Leg Treading Plié Squeeze Leg Lunge	_____ _____ _____
	Shake Out		
	Combination:	The Butterflyer Pendulum Body Swing	_____ _____
COOL-DOWN (5 min.)	Leg Split Cross Chest Stretch Head Circles		_____ _____ _____

WEEK 8

Your W.E.T. workout now has three combination exercises. Keep up the great work!

Comments:

WARM-UP (5 min.)	**Water Walking** **Aqua Lunge** **Arm Stretch**		_____ _____ _____
W.E.T. SET (15 min.)	**Upper:**	**Rear Push-Ups** **Sport Arm Pump** **Medley of Strokes**	_____ _____ _____
	Shake Out		
	Middle:	**Circle Spray** **Sit-Ups** **Body Wave**	_____ _____ _____
	Shake Out		
	Lower:	**Leg Crossover** **Medley of Kicks** **Aqua Dancer**	_____ _____ _____
	Shake Out		
	Combination:	**The Freestyler** **The Sidestroker** **Aqua Jumping Jacks**	_____ _____ _____
COOL-DOWN (5 min.)	**Standing Tall** **Runner's Calf Stretch** **Overhead Stretch**		_____ _____ _____

WEEK 9

Now that your conditioning has improved, your W.E.T. set increases to 20 minutes. Let's do each W.E.T. for 1½ minutes.

Comments:

WARM-UP (5 min.)	**Toe Tester** **Head Circles** **Shoulder Shrug**		_____ _____ _____
W.E.T. SET (20 min.— 1½ minutes per exercise)	**Upper:**	**Hang "10"** **Sport Swings** **Scull and Hug**	_____ _____ _____
	Shake Out		
	Middle:	**Back Extension** **Sit-Ups** **Trunk Twist**	_____ _____ _____
	Shake Out		
	Lower:	**Plié Squeeze** **Rockette Kick** **Leg Treading**	_____ _____ _____
	Shake Out		
	Combination:	**The Backstroker** **Pendulum Body Swing** **Ballet V**	_____ _____ _____
COOL-DOWN (5 min.)	**Cross Chest Stretch** **Runner's Quadriceps Stretch** **Standing Tall**		_____ _____ _____

WEEK 10

Increase the time for each W.E.T., e.g. 1½ min. each.

WARM-UP
(5 min.)
Water Walking
Triceps Stretch
Ballet Leg Stretch

W.E.T. SET
(20 min.)

Upper:	Push-Ups	(1 min.)
	Medley of Strokes	(1½ min.)
	Water Push	(2 min.)

Shake Out

Middle:	Knee Tuck	(1 min.)
	Sit-Ups	(1½ min.)
	Circle Spray	(2 min.)

Shake Out

Lower:	Leg Lunge	(1 min.)
	Medley of Kicks	(1½ min.)
	Leg Swirl	(2 min.)

Shake Out

Combination:	The Butterflyer	(1 min.)
	Treading	(1½ min.)
	Aqua Jumping Jacks	(2 min.)

COOL-DOWN
(5 min.)
Head Circles
Shoulder Shrug
Pike Body Stretch

WEEK 11

Vary the intensity of your W.E.T. set with "Fartlek" training: work for 30 seconds easy, then 30 seconds hard, then 30 seconds moderate. This interval training originated in Sweden. Repeat each W.E.T. in this manner.

Comments:

WARM-UP (5 min.)	**Water Walking** **Shoulder Shrug with "Chicken Wings"** **Aqua Lunge**		_____ _____ _____
W.E.T. SET (20 min.)	**Upper:**	**Rear Push-Ups** **Arm and Wrist Swirls** **Sculling**	_____ _____ _____
	Shake Out		
	Middle:	**Corner Leg Swing** **Hip Touch** **Body Wave**	_____ _____ _____
	Shake Out		
	Lower:	**Leg Treading** **Leg Swirl** **Leg Crossover**	_____ _____ _____
	Shake Out		
	Combination:	**The Breaststroker** **Treading** **The Sidestroker**	_____ _____ _____
COOL-DOWN (5 min.)	**Cross Chest Stretch** **Ballet Leg Stretch** **Toe Tester with "Crossover"**		_____ _____ _____

WEEK 12

Add quantity to your quality. Now there are four W.E.T.s for each body area. Keep up your W.E.T. program to maintain your newfound fitness. This expanded workout may take 30—45 minutes to complete.

Comments:

WARM-UP **Overhead Stretch** _____
(5 min.) **Water Walking** _____
   Pike Body Stretch _____
   Standing Tall _____

W.E.T. SET **Upper:** **Sport Arm Pump** _____
(20—30 min.)   **Water Push** _____
      Sport Swings _____
      Rear Push-Ups _____
   Shake Out
   Middle: **Back Extension** _____
      Buttock Squeeze _____
      Circle Spray _____
      Overhead Swing _____
   Shake Out
   Lower: **Leg Lunge** _____
      Rockette Kick _____
      Medley of Kicks _____
      Aqua Dancer _____
   Shake Out
   Combination: **The Backstroker** _____
      Ballet V _____
      Coordinated Sport Arm _____
        and Leg Motions
      The Freestyler (with breathing) _____

COOL-DOWN **Leg Split** _____
(5 min.) **Runner's Quadriceps Stretch** _____
   Arm Stretch _____
   Standing Tall _____

WEEK 13 AND BEYOND

It's up to you to keep maintaining your F.I.T.ness with your W.E.T. workouts. Copy this page, and mix 'n' match to create your own W.E.T. workout combinations! See following chapters for additional suggestions.

W.E.T. PROGRESSIVE WORKOUT LOG   Comments:

WARM-UP   _____   _____
(5 min.)   _____   _____
                               _____   _____

W.E.T. SET   Upper:_____   _____
(20–30 min.)   _____   _____
                               _____   _____

                  Shake Out

                  Middle: _____   _____
                               _____   _____
                               _____   _____

                  Shake Out

                  Lower: _____   _____
                               _____   _____
                               _____   _____

                  Shake Out

                  Combination: _____   _____
                               _____   _____
                               _____   _____

COOL-DOWN   _____   _____
(5 min.)   _____   _____
                               _____   _____

CHARTING YOUR W.E.T. WORKOUT: PERSONAL LOG

MAIN W.E.T. SET

Month	Week	Day	Warm-Up	Upper	Middle	Lower	Combination	Cool-Down	Total	Comments
1	1									
	2									
	3									
	4									

(continued on following page)

MAIN W.E.T. SET (continued)

Month	Week	Day	Warm-Up	Upper	Middle	Lower	Combination	Cool-Down	Total	Comments
2	5									
	6									
	7									
	8									
3	9									
	10									
	11									
	12									

W.E.T.s with Equipment

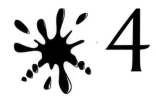

4

This chapter highlights water exercises that use aquatic equipment, which can be divided into categories of traditional swim equipment, specific water exercise equipment, and additional aquatic exercise equipment. The chapter concludes with a sample "circuit training workout" that combines several applications.

Traditional Swim Equipment

Conventional swimming equipment can also be used for water exercise. Among the most common and popular are kickboards, hand paddles, pull-buoys, and fins.

Using this equipment increases resistance of individual exercises, enhances enjoyment through variety, increases the intensity of a workout (i.e., fat burning), and maximizes fun.

The Kickboard

Kickboards are a basic swim training device. They are made of buoyant materials and are designed to lift and stabilize the arms and upper body during kicking drills. Their size and shape make them very useful for water exercises. In addition, kickboards with openings are available specifically for water exercise and provide variable resistance.

EQUIPMENT TIP

Kickboards are available in most aquatic facilities. There are additional kickboard W.E.T.s in chapter 7 on page 120.

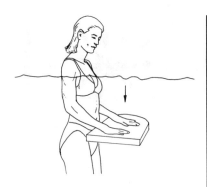

KICKBOARD PRESSES

Starting Position: Stand in chest-deep water with your hands on a kickboard held widthwise.

Technique:
1. Slowly straighten your arms and push the board downward under the water.
2. Slowly allow the board to return to the surface.

OCEAN IN A POOL

Starting Position: Stand in chest-deep water and hold kickboard widthwise, perpendicular to the water's surface.

Technique: Bring board close to body, submerged as much as possible. Extend your arms, pushing water and board away from the body. Then bring board quickly toward chest and repeat. Do this exercise with a lot of energy, leaning your body into each movement, alternating the board in each direction to maximize wave action.

Variation: "Kickboard Waterfall": In chest-deep water, hold the board widthwise flat on the water's surface with arms extended forward. Submerge the board, and then lift board and water until arms are extended overhead to create a waterfall.

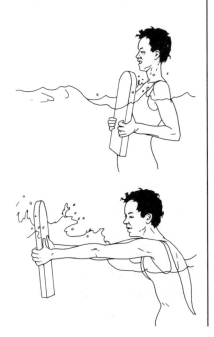

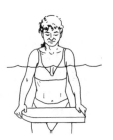

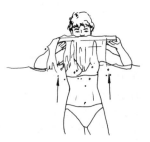

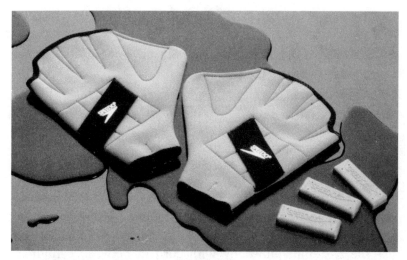

Hand Paddles, Mitts, and Gloves

Hand paddles are one of the most common pieces of swimming equipment and can be found in a variety of colors and styles; mitts also come in a variety of colors, styles, and thicknesses. They are most commonly used to increase resistance when you simulate a stroke, such as the crawl stroke.

Before exercising with the equipment, try a resistance check. Place the mitt or hand paddle on your hand; slide your arm forward and back from your elbow just under the surface of the water, with hand parallel to the surface of the water. You should not feel much resistance. If you press your hand under water, you can feel more water resistance by flexing your hand upward and downward.

ARM SCULL AND CLAP

Starting Position: Stand in chest-deep water with arms underwater, extended in front of body, wearing hand paddles, mitts, or webbed gloves.

Technique: Sweep arms out to sides with palms facing outward. Continue to sweep arms as far as possible until they touch or approach each

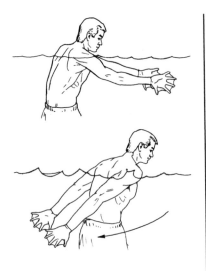

other behind body; then reverse palms toward front of body and sweep arms forward to meet again in front of chest.

Variation: Walk, slide, or leap in various directions for a more energetic exercise.

Pull-Buoy

Pull-buoys are usually made of buoyant Styrofoam material and are primarily used for swim training. You can use pull-buoys in W.E.T.s to help develop strength as your muscles resist the upward buoyant force which the water exerts on the pull-buoy. Use the treadmill pull-buoy with cord in between cylindrical buoys.

SIDE SWIPE

Starting Position: Stand in waist- to chest-deep water, holding on to the pool edge or corner with both arms. Place foot on pull-buoy, or use an ankle cuff.

Technique: Begin at water's surface with leg extended to the side. Sweep leg down and in front of body in semicircular pattern and then return to starting position. Remember to keep hips as even as possible. Begin with several sweeps on each side (e.g., five). Remove cuff or pull-buoy, replace on other leg, and repeat on other side, being sure to do an equal number of sweeps on each side.

Variation: "Rockette Kick": Add a pull-buoy under your heel. More effort is required because of the buoyancy of the pull-buoy. You can also use a buoyancy/resistance "cuff" for this exercise.

Fins

For many years fins have been standard gear for skin and scuba divers, and have now entered the swimmers' arena where they are used for the teaching of skills, aerobic conditioning, general fitness, and workout variety. They have also become popular among water exercisers as a training tool because of the increased water resistance that exercises the large leg muscles more vigorously.

Unlike the utilitarian look of the standard heavy, flat diver's fin, current state-of-the-art fin technology and design offer swimmers of all levels a range of styles, materials, weight, color, size, fit, and comfort.

QUADRICEPS STRETCH

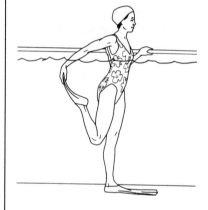

Starting Position: Stand in waist- to chest-deep water, with knees together, wearing fins and holding on to pool edge with one hand for support, as needed.

Technique: Bending one knee, bring foot as close to buttocks as possible. Then, allowing knees to separate, grasp end of fin and continue to bring foot toward buttocks. Feel the stretch in front of thigh. Release and repeat on other side.

HAMSTRING/THIGH CHALLENGE

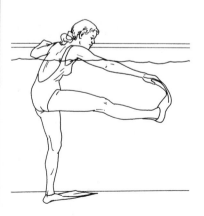

Starting Position: Stand in waist-deep water perpendicular to the pool edge, wearing fins and holding on to the edge of the pool.

Technique: With your outside hand, grasp the tip of the fin on the outside leg, and lift that leg so that your hamstrings as well as inner and outer thigh muscles are stretched. Move the leg outward to the side and then forward. Release, turn around, and stretch your other leg.

SIT 'N' KICK WITH FINS

Starting Position: Sit on pool edge with feet in water, wearing fins.

Technique: Drop your heels to the wall; then simultaneously straighten your knees and lift your legs to the water's surface. Repeat.

Specific W.E.T. Equipment

Equipment is also made specifically for water exercise. Following are examples of exercises that utilize them.

Paddles and Wands

PADDLE PLANES

Starting Position: Stand in shoulder- to chest-deep water, holding resistance device underwater.

Technique: Move arms through the water. Vary the resistance against which the arms move by changing planes of movement. For example, using a "slicing" movement gives little resistance; moving against direction of arm motion with the widest plane of the device provides greatest resistance.

Variation:	If using adjustable wands, experiment with the open and closed positions, varying resistance as you exercise.

PADDLE SPORTS SWING

Starting Position:	Stand in chest-deep water, holding resistance device underwater.
Technique:	Practice sweeping/swinging arm underwater. Can be used to enhance sports swing or for arm/shoulder exercise.
Equipment:	Wands, Aqua Flex paddles.
Variation:	Combine with walk or slide movement through water.

Buoyancy/Resistance Cuffs for Ankles and/or Wrists

DEEP WATER JUMPING JACKS

Starting Position:	Stand in chin-deep water, with arms extended to the side and legs in straddle position.
Technique:	Simultaneously and vigorously bring arms to sides and legs together, causing body to rise out of water, into a soldier's stance. Then return to starting position.
Variation:	Cross arms and/or legs left over right.

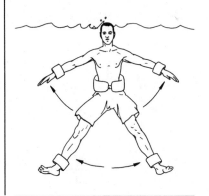

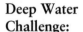
Deep Water Challenge:

Reverse the position. Starting in vertical streamlined position, simultaneously and vigorously extend arms out to sides and separate legs. You will be working against the buoyancy and resistance of the cuffs. Be prepared for possible submerging of face (for a moment). Then bring arms down and legs together to return to starting position.

Barbells

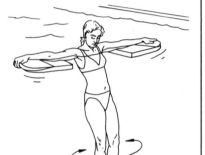

HELICOPTER

Starting Position:

In deep water begin in vertical position with arms extended to the sides holding flotation devices. Keep legs straight and together, and ankles crossed.

Technique:

Rotate legs from the waist, sweeping them to the right, back, and left, and then return to the streamlined vertical position. Repeat in the opposite direction.

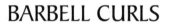

BARBELL CURLS

Starting Position:

Standing in shoulder- to neck-deep water, hold barbell in either or both hands, with arms extended downward toward thighs.

Technique:

Curl arms upward, keeping elbows close to body. Bring barbell up to surface of the water *slowly*, working against the buoyancy of the barbells. Then bring barbells back down to sides, working against the resistance and the buoyancy of the water.

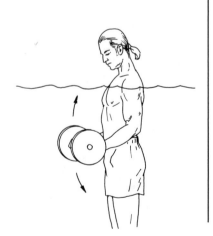

Variation:	If you are using two barbells, you can turn palms in opposite directions: one facing downward and one facing upward. On subsequent repetitions, change direction of hands.

DEEP WATER SIT-UPS

Starting Position:	Begin from back float with feet together, arms extended to the side, using flotation devices.
Technique:	Draw knees toward chest, and then straighten legs. (Buttocks will lower into water while knees are bent.)
Equipment:	Kickboards, water-wing floaters, flotation cuffs, foam barbells, log.
Variation:	Practice sit-up in prone float position with arms extended in front of body holding flotation devices. Draw knees to chest, then return to floating position by straightening legs.

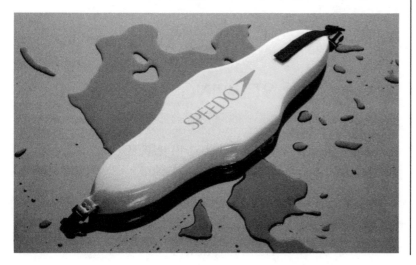

W.E.T. TIP

Barbell curls are an example of an exercise which uses the antagonistic muscle groups of biceps and triceps.

EQUIPMENT TIP

There is also a piece of equipment that is a cross between a barbell and a rowing oar. The ends are designed with removable paddles with several large surface areas (blades) to work against the water's resistance.

EQUIPMENT TIP

Flotation belts provide neutral buoyancy for safety and comfort. Please see box on page 101.

Flotation Belts and Vests

COSSACK KICK

Starting Position: Stand in shoulder- to neck-deep water, or floating vertically in streamlined position in deep water. Arms are underwater.

Technique: Lift legs into straddle position simultaneously with feet kicking outward.

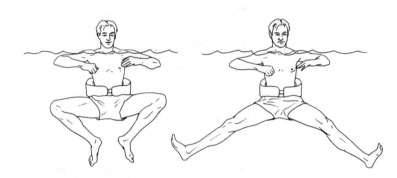

Aquatic Step

STEPPING

Starting Position: Stand in chest-deep water four to six inches in front of the aquatic step, which is width-wise in front of you.

Technique: Start using the aquatic step by alternately "stepping" up and down on it. Start with the right foot leading, i.e., right, left, up; right, left, down.

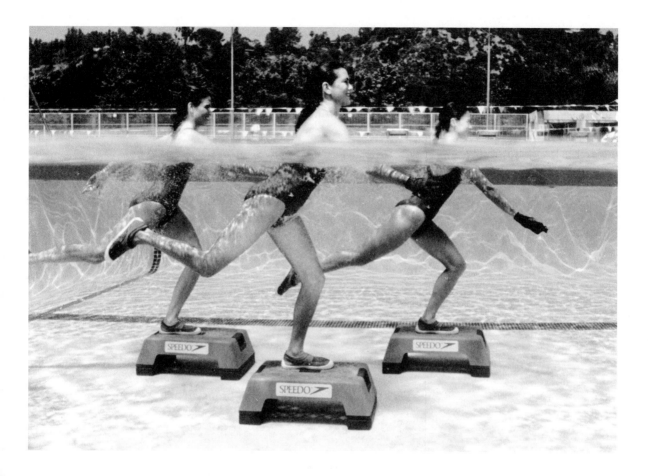

ROCKING HORSE

Starting Position: Stand in chest-deep water, about four to eight inches from aquatic step.

Technique: Moving with an alternate forward and backward motion, step or rock onto the step with lead foot and then return to starting position. Then rock onto step again and bring your other foot onto the top of the step. Rock down to the other side of the step. Turn 180° to face step again and repeat on other side using other leg to lead.

W.E.T. TIP

Place feet at center of step. Use sculling hand movements for balance and support.

DEEP WATER SIT-UPS WITH LOG

Starting Position: Start from back float position, with feet together, arms extended to the side, grasping log.

Technique: Draw knee toward chest, and then straighten legs (buttocks will lower into the water while knees are bent).

BREASTSTROKE SWIM WITH LOG (NOODLE)

Starting Position: Place log under armpits and float in water.

Technique: Practice breaststroke arm motion with or without leg kick.

Tethered Exercise

Tethered swimming is simply attaching a rope to a swimmer from a stationary point on the pool deck, which allows him to swim in place. The advantage of tethered exercise is that it makes swimming or water jogging possible in a small pool or a large spa.

Tethers have come a long way. Decades ago, swimmers trained using a rope attached to their waist to keep them stationary as they pulled, kicked or swam. Now tethered exercise is done by attaching an elastic band—often a stretch cord—and having the swimmer move as far out into the pool as possible. An extra training benefit comes from working against the additional resistance (the pull of the cord as well as that of the water). The swimmer develops muscles and cardiovascular fitness by "fighting" for a few more yards into the pool.

A variation is to do tethered exercise against a water flow, or flume.

Tethered exercise can be used either for swim strokes or deep-water jogging/running. Be certain that the tether is attached to the deck as close as possible to the water's surface for tethered water jogging. In the case of fiberglass rods (similar to a fishing pole!), the rod will flex as the swimmer "swims" out into the pool away from the wall. The tether can be attached to the waist, wrists, ankles, or feet (with special shoes).

When jogging in place use more power, as if you are jogging uphill, moving away from the wall. When you jog with less energy, you will be close to the wall.

Large Stationary Equipment

Water Workout Station

There are large, versatile, stationary water workout stations available for poolside placement that include steps, rails, platform extensions, etc., to challenge the water exerciser. An example of their use is included here.

WORKOUT STATION STRETCH

Starting Position:	Float on back, holding onto ladder or other pool structure.
Technique:	Straighten legs and extend out from ladder. Then swing from side to side by bending alternate arms, moving body in direction of bent arm.

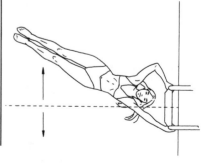

Water Treadmill

Water treadmills allow an exerciser to actively walk or jog underwater. Water treadmills can vary both speed and incline, which can be regulated to suit the exercise needs of the aqua runner. Distance and speed can be measured using a digital display; safety is enhanced by handrails and an emergency stop button, similar to those on "dry" treadmills. These familiar features make the water treadmill user-friendly to many water exercisers.

The workout consists of applying the F.I.T. principle by progressively increasing speed as well as grade to provide aerobic training. Wearing aqua shoes or waterproof sneakers on the water treadmill is recommended.

Sample Water Treadmill Set
3 min. easy walking (e.g., 2.0 to 3.5 mph)
3 min. moderate jog (e.g., 4.0 mph)
1 min. easy jog
2 min. fast jog
1 min. easy jog

Vary the grade (incline) for greater or less effort.

Circuit Training

An aquatic training circuit includes different exercises using various equipment, which are placed in stations throughout the pool. Beginning at one station, the exerciser practices for a set period of time (e.g., 5 minutes) and then moves to the next station. The workout is completed when the exerciser returns to the starting station.

Each piece of equipment we've discussed can also be used in circuit training. Circuit training is an ideal exercise program for group participation as well as for athletes who wish to maintain fitness levels in the off season, rehabilitate injuries in any season, or add variety to regular practice sessions. Circuits can also be used for cross training.

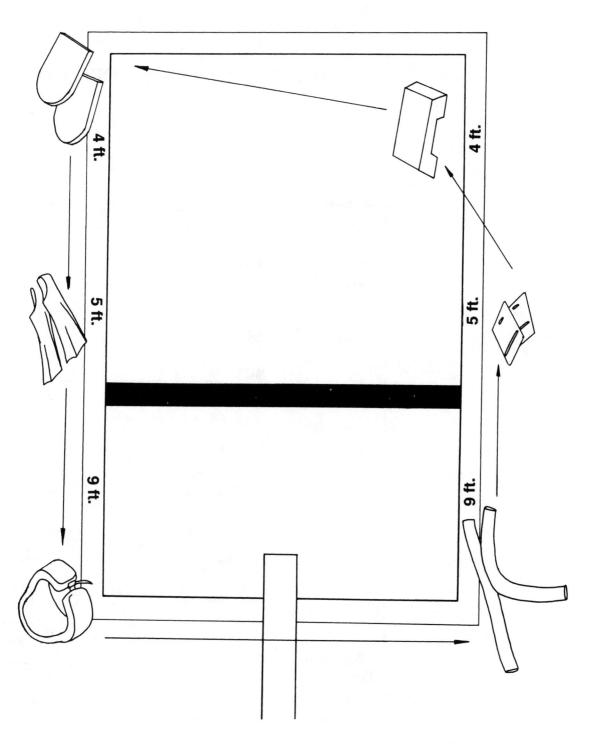

CREATE YOUR OWN
W.E.T. EQUIPMENT WORKOUT

EQUIPMENT W.E.T. WORKOUT LOG

Time and/or
repetitions

WARM-UP
(5 min.)
_____ _____
_____ _____
_____ _____

W.E.T. SET   Upper:_____ _____
(10–30 min.)
_____ _____
_____ _____

Shake Out

Middle: _____ _____
_____ _____
_____ _____

Shake Out

Lower: _____ _____
_____ _____
_____ _____

Shake Out

Combination:_____ _____
_____ _____
_____ _____

COOL-DOWN   _____ _____
(5 min.)
_____ _____
_____ _____

Sport Cross Training W.E.T.s

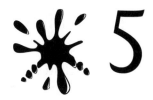

Those were the days—the medicine ball days! The smelly gyms, with sweaty people throwing medicine balls. But long before the term "rehab" and "cross training" were popular, "real" athletes simply called it "training." For seasonal players, cross training was a way to maximize the aerobic effect of their conditioning and minimize downtime from injury. Coaches used cross training to avoid overuse injury among their players; professional players cross-trained to prolong their careers.

For many athletes, cross-training regimens in the water often begin during a period of rehabilitation after an injury, or often as a preventive measure against overuse damage. Cross-training W.E.T.s have many benefits:

- ❑ the increased resistance of the water strengthens muscles; water's uniform resistance is an added plus
- ❑ decreased shocking of joints provides the opportunity to train virtually injury-free
- ❑ water slows motion down so that you can concentrate on sport-specific movements

The aim of this chapter is to help athletes train for their chosen sport by cross-training with W.E.T.s. It outlines basic locomotor movements in the water and applies them first to the major fitness activities of walking and running, and then to a variety of other popular sports. You can develop your personal W.E.T. cross-

> **Plyometrics** is the use of elastic energy and recoil similar to that seen in springboard diving, or a gymnast's flight through the air from a "beat board." Plyometrics is intrinsic to jumping and rebounding movements, and can be applied to basic locomotor skills in the water. Its buoyant properties allow you to focus on the height of your "jump" and distance through the water.

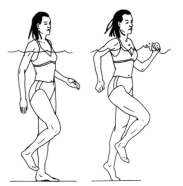

Walking   Jogging

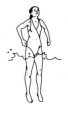

Jumping

training program as a seasonal training tool, which can be tailored to meet your needs.

Whether your W.E.T. workout is the core of your training program, or you cross-train by using the water as one part of your complete fitness-conditioning regimen, the water will help you attain your sport or fitness goals.

Water Walking and Locomotor W.E.T.s

Locomotor Skills

Remember childhood games of hopscotch and jump rope? These are examples of basic locomotive movements that can be trans-

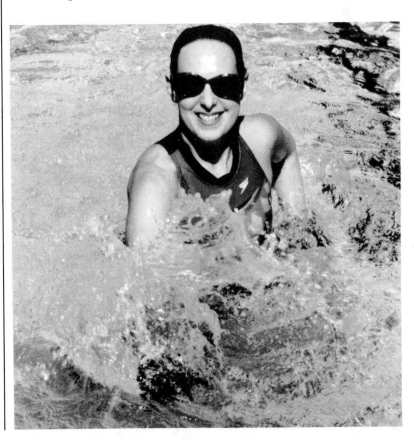

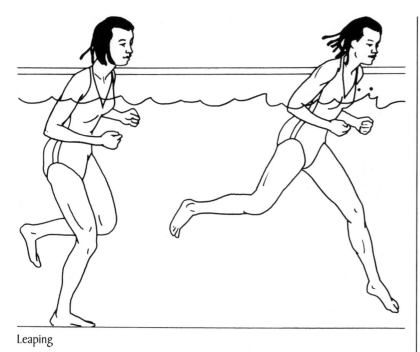

Leaping

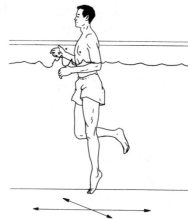

Hopping

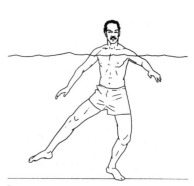

Lunging

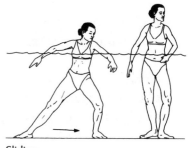

Sliding

ferred into the water. These skills can be practiced initially in place, and then moving forward, backward, sideways, diagonally, and in a circular pattern.

Walking—placing one foot in front of the other, as on land, with arms moving in opposition to legs (i.e., left foot forward, right hand forward). In the water, walking will be slower than on land because of the resistance of the water. You can begin walking in place with a marching step, and then progress to fast walking and into a jog.

Jumping—moving the body from the ground simultaneously using both legs. The "shake out" between exercises (see page 50) is really a plyometric jump.

Jump Locomotor Skill: Begin standing in chest-deep water. Lift legs simultaneously off pool bottom, allowing the buoyancy of the water to suspend body. Move forward or backward by adjusting angle of foot against pool bottom.

From water walking you can intensify your workout into a race walk, and then into shallow-water running. Every 15 seconds, change speeds. For example:

1. walking   (15 secs.)
2. race walking   (15 secs.)
3. shallow water running (15 secs.)

Rest 15 seconds and repeat set.

LOCOMOTOR W.E.T. COMBINATIONS

Use arms for balance and propulsion for locomotor W.E.T.s.

Add locomotor moves together: for example, combine jogging in place with Water Pushes. Or move across the pool walking, then sliding, hopping, jumping, etc.

Another variation is to use locomotor W.E.T.s with other exercises. After each locomotor crossing of the pool, flutter kick on the wall for 30 seconds, or do 10 water Push-Ups. Also, break up your lap by adding 5 to 10 Jumping Aqua Jacks when you have moved to the middle of the pool.

Hopping—moving the body off the ground using one foot and landing on the same foot. Repeat on other foot.

Hop Locomotor Skill: Raise one knee toward chest. Use remaining foot to jump off pool bottom. Move forward, backward, left, or right by changing angle of foot as it leaves pool bottom.

Lunging—Alternately extend one leg out to the side while bending the other.

Skipping—a forward hop on alternate feet with a step in between each hop.

Sliding—moving in a given direction, keeping constant contact with the surface, with one foot leading and the other foot following.

Locomotor Skill Slide: Begin standing with feet together and arms at sides. Extend one foot outward to side, using arms to maintain balance in the water. Bring second foot to extended foot, moving body in direction of first extension.

Leaping—lifting the body suddenly from the floor, starting on one foot and landing on the other; for example, a "rocking horse" exercise forward and back.

ROCKING HORSE LEAP

Starting Position: Stand in chest-deep water with one leg in front of the other, and weight on back leg.

Technique: Rock forward onto front leg, trying to gain height during the leap. Then rock backward, returning to rear leg. Do several times on one leg and then reverse front legs.

These movements can be put together into many combinations, such as step, hop, and jump.

SAMPLE WALKING AND LOCOMOTOR W.E.T. WORKOUT

WARM-UP

Warm-Up W.E.T.s	5 minutes

MAIN SET

Water Walking—Easy	5 minutes
Jumps and Leaps	1 minute
Water Walking—Easy to Moderate	4 minutes
Leaps and Sliding	1 minute
Water Walking—Moderate	3 minutes
Hops	1 minute
Water Walking—Moderate to Fast	2 minutes
Leaps	1 minute
Water Walking	1 minute

COOL-DOWN

Cool Down W.E.T.s	5 minutes

CREATE YOUR OWN
W.E.T. LOCOMOTOR WORKOUT

W.E.T. WORKOUT LOG

Comments: e.g., time
and/or repetitions

WARM-UP
(5 min.)
_____ _____
_____ _____
_____ _____

W.E.T. SET
(10–30 min.)
_____ _____
_____ _____
_____

Shake Out

_____ _____
_____ _____
_____ _____

Shake Out

_____ _____
_____ _____
_____ _____

Shake Out

Combination:_____ _____
_____ _____
_____ _____

COOL-DOWN _____ _____
(5 min.) _____ _____
_____ _____

Sport W.E.T.s

This section is designed for the serious athlete who wishes to cross-train in the water. The basic movements of over a dozen sports have been isolated for a water environment to help teach and reinforce technique, while strengthening and/or stretching muscles for improved performance. A good way to make the most of training in the water is to first observe an elite athlete in your sport. Then isolate techniques that you wish to reinforce. Practice the skill on land (perhaps watching in a mirror so you can see yourself move). Then transfer the skill to water and incorporate it into your W.E.T. workout.

The "killer W.E.T.s" are vigorous sets that can be incorporated into the main set of a water workout for experienced, well-conditioned athletes.

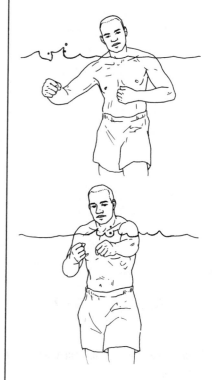

Training seasons for various sports usually are divided into three parts, each about 8–12 weeks in length.

❑ early season
❑ mid-season
❑ peak season (for events)

BOXING PUNCHES

Starting Position: Stand in chest-deep water with feet in boxing stance.

Technique: Practice boxing technique:
Jab—Punch arms forward from body.
Hook—Swing either arm around from the side.
Undercut—Begin arm swing with elbow bent, starting from waist. Extend arm upward to water's surface, straightening elbow.

Equipment: Mitts or buoyancy cuffs optional.

Killer W.E.T. Set: Pyramid: 2–3–4–3–2
2 Jabs, 2 Hooks, 2 Undercuts, 2 Karate Kicks
Rest and Shake Out
3 Jabs, 3 Hooks, 3 Undercuts, 3 Karate Kicks
Rest and Shake Out
4 Jabs, 4 Hooks, 4 Undercuts, 4 Karate

Kicks
Rest and Shake Out
3 Jabs, 3 Hooks, 3 Undercuts, 3 Karate
Kicks
Rest and Shake Out
2 Jabs, 2 Hooks, 2 Undercuts, 2 Karate
Kicks
(Optional: Boxing shuffle between sets)

GYMNASTIC/ICE SKATING ARABESQUE

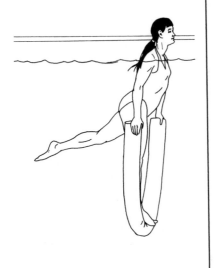

Starting Position: Stand in chest-deep water with arms extended to your sides.

Technique: Raise leg behind body, maintaining balance. Keep leg straight and raise as high as possible. Return leg to pool bottom and raise other leg.

Equipment: Log, kickboard.

Variation: Use log to do this exercise in deep water. Hold onto ends of log while balancing on log. A kickboard is a further challenge to your balance.

Killer W.E.T. Set: Hold balance for incremental periods starting at 5 and ending at 30 seconds for each leg. Change sides by swinging leg over top of log, in front of body.

DOWNHILL SKI MOGULS

Starting Position: Stand in chest-deep water to one side of the stripe that marks out the lanes. (Use a similar stationary landmark on the pool bottom if the lane stripe is not available.)

Technique:	Jump with knees bent upward chest to clear the mogul (pool stripe). Press arms and hands down against the water to gain height.

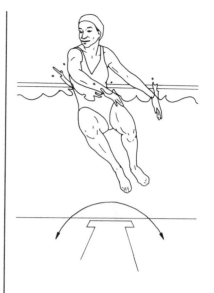

Killer W.E.T. Set: Descending Pyramid: 2 x 8–6–4–2
8 jumps facing pool wall, ½ turn
8 jumps facing pool, ½ turn
6 jumps facing pool wall, ½ turn
6 jumps facing pool, ½ turn
4 jumps facing pool wall, ½ turn
4 jumps facing pool, ½ turn
2 jumps facing pool wall, ½ turn
2 jumps facing pool, ½ turn

Option: Repeat set.

CROSS-COUNTRY SKIING

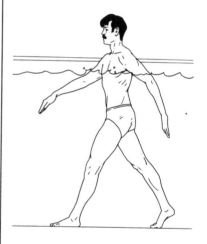

Starting Position: Stand in chest-deep water with legs shoulder width apart.

Technique: Extend one arm forward in front of body, and the leg on that side behind body. Extend the other arm behind body, and extend the leg on that side forward. Jump and alternate forward and backward motion, with arms and legs moving in opposition to each other, maintaining equal strides.

Equipment: Water shoes recommended; hand paddles/mitts optional

Variation: Cross-country ski in deep water, using flotation device for greater buoyancy.

Killer W.E.T. Set: **Descending/Ascending Pyramid Set with ¼ turn for direction change:**

8 strides facing to the front, ¼ turn
8 strides facing to the right, ¼ turn
8 strides facing to the back, ¼ turn
8 strides facing to the left, ¼ turn
6 strides facing to the front, ¼ turn
6 strides facing to the right, ¼ turn
Etc., etc.

ROLLER BLADING

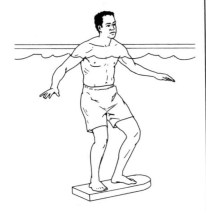

Starting Position: In deep water, stand on log or kickboard.

Technique: Bend and straighten knees, maintaining balance.

Equipment: Log, preferably shorter than standard size or kickboard.

Variation: Practice maintaining balance for 15 seconds, then increase time to 30 seconds, then 1 minute at a time.

Killer W.E.T. Set: **With kickboard**
Bend and straighten knees as fast as you can without falling off the kickboard!

HURDLES

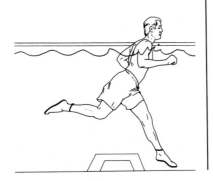

Starting Position: Standing in chest-deep water.

Technique: Simulate a hurdle running movement. Begin with your knees together under your body. Then your front leg extends straight forward, and your rear leg is bent behind you.

Return to the standing position; turn around and repeat with opposite leg forward.

Equipment: Aquatic step.

Variation: Practice clearing the step, first width-wise, then lengthwise.

Killer W.E.T. Set: Practice hurdle movement backwards.

SPORTS SWING

Starting Position: Stand in chest-deep water.

Technique: Practice appropriate swing for chosen sport, e.g., tennis, golf, baseball, squash, etc. Hold both arms together and follow through swing, paying attention to correct mechanics of chosen sport.

Equipment: Hand paddles or mitts optional.

Killer W.E.T. Set: 10 reps both arms
10 reps right arm
10 reps left arm
Shake Out
10 reps with weaker arm

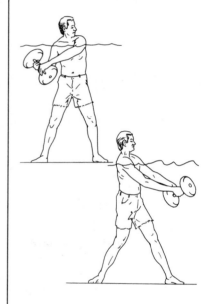

FOOTBALL

Starting Position: Standing in shallow water.

Technique: Run in place using short strides and short arm motions.

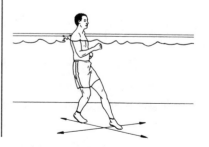

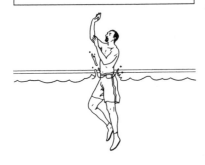

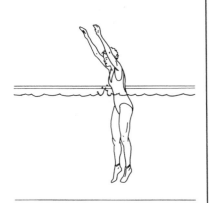

Killer W.E.T. Set:	Practice the football scramble, moving forward, backward, to the right, and to the left.

BASKETBALL JUMP FOR HEIGHT

Starting Position:	Stand in shoulder- to chest-deep water.
Technique:	Jump out of the water with a plyometric movement, as if shooting a basketball.
Equipment:	Aqua shoes.
Killer W.E.T. Set:	Alternate right hand, left hand, both hands. Dribble for 10 seconds in between each.

VOLLEYBALL SPIKE

Starting Position:	Stand in chest-deep water in volleyball stance.
Technique:	Practice a height jump with a plyometric movement, as when spiking the ball. Remember to get your hips up.
Equipment:	Aqua shoes
Killer W.E.T. Set:	Practice left, right, and two-handed spikes in succession.

SOCCER KICK

Starting Position: Stand in chest-deep water.

Technique: Practice soccer kick; extend leg forcefully, varying foot position; alternating right and left leg.

Equipment: Aqua shoes.

Killer W.E.T. Set: Jog and Soccer Kick: Practice soccer kick "around the clock": Kick at "12 o'clock," jog 6 steps, kick at "1 o'clock," jog 6 steps, etc.

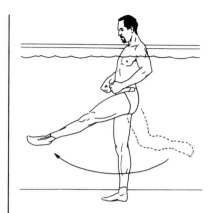

DANCE LEG LIFT

Starting Position: Stand in chest-deep water, holding kickboard width-wise.

Technique: Raise leg, extending it forward with knee straight. Maintain balance and keep body vertical and streamlined. Return leg to bottom and repeat on other side.

Equipment: Kickboard, log. Aqua shoes optional.

Variation: Move leg out to side.

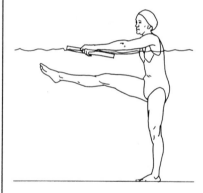

ARCHERY

Starting Position: Standing in chest-deep water with arms underwater.

Technique: Practice archery extension, holding bands or stretch cords, keeping arms below water's surface.

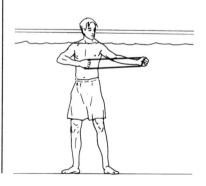

Equipment:	Elastic tubing, stretch cords.
Variation:	Use tether.

DIVING APPROACH: THREE STEPS AND HURDLE

Starting Position:	Stand in waist- to chest-deep water at cross-bar of lane stripe of bottom of pool. Determine starting point by measuring the three steps plus hurdle distance, as you would while diving.
Technique:	Take three steps and hurdle; jump forward to "clear" the pool stripe (diving board). Keep body streamlined. Walk back to starting point and repeat.
Equipment:	Aqua shoes.

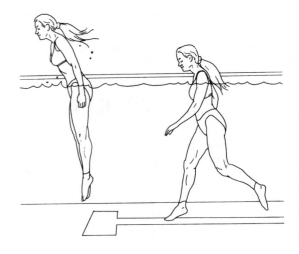

WEIGHTLIFTING TRICEPS KICKBOARD PRESS

W.E.T. TIP

Bring shoulder blades as close as possible together. Use 2 or more boards for greater challenge.

Starting Position: Stand in chest-deep water, with shoulder blades back and chest forward. Hold kickboard behind your body in vertical position with curved edge (if any) upward. Face your elbows outward and hold the board close to your body.

Technique: Extend your arms downward, pressing the board downward as far as possible against the buoyancy of the water. Then bend elbows slowly to return the board back to starting position, being careful to control the kickboard.

Variation: For greater resistance, turn board widthwise and press away from body.

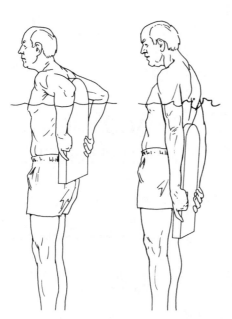

DOUBLE BOARD PRESS

Starting Position: Float in vertical position in deep water, holding a standard kickboard under each arm.

Technique: Simultaneously press boards downward against the resistance of the water.

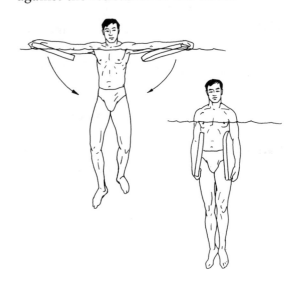

AQUATIC STEP CHALLENGE

Starting Position: Stand in chest- to shoulder-deep water, holding onto the sides of an aquatic step, with the flat surface next to your chest.

Technique: With step just at water's surface, alternately push step forward and back using water's resistance.

Deep Water Running W.E.T.s

Ask deep water runners why they are in the pool, and the two most common answers will be that (a) they are runners who are recovering from an injury and want to keep moving during the rehabilitation period, and (b) they began deep water running as rehabilitation exercise, and now retain it as a complement to their restored running program.

Deep water running meets the needs of a wide range of participants—marathoners, triathletes, as well as cross trainers. Vertical deep water exercise provides these athletes with specificity of training and maintenance of their aerobic conditioning while preventing overuse injury. Deep water running also provides an alternative fitness regiment for major athletes concerned about extending their professional careers. It is also helpful to the arthritis patient, who can move more freely in the water, as well as to the "average person" who is looking for a pleasant, effective way to keep in shape.

RUNNING INJURIES

Charles Greene, 1968 Olympic track and field gold medalist in the 4 x 100 meter relay and the 1996 Olympic assistant track and field coach for the 4 x 100 meter relay, explains common runner's injuries:

❑ Shin splints are usually caused by the foot impacting the ground. Stretching and icing after running are crucial to injury prevention and healing.

❑ Hamstring and groin injuries are frequently caused by lack of stretching or failure to warm up properly.

Greene says that a water exercise program can be helpful for full recovery from such injuries, because it eliminates the stress on the body's musculoskeletal system.

DEEP WATER RUNNING

Technique:	Run as you do on land, paying attention to your form. Keep your elbows close to your body, moving your arms in opposition to your legs. Maintain your body posture.
Equipment:	Flotation belt.
Variation:	Do tether running backward, keeping arms underwater.

DEEP WATER CHALLENGE SET

Warm up: 5 min.

Main W.E.T. Set:

Four 30-second runs with 15 second rest intervals in each of four different strides. 1 min. recovery run between each.

- ❏ power walking
- ❏ long strides
- ❏ uphill with knee lift
- ❏ downhill run with short stride

- ❏ 3 min.–2 min.–1 min.–30 sec. without any break. Increase cadence with each increment

Cool down: 5 min.

CREATE YOUR OWN SPORT CROSS-TRAINING W.E.T. WORKOUT

W.E.T. WORKOUT LOG

Comments: e.g., time
and/or repetitions

WARM-UP
(5 min.)

_____   _____
_____   _____
_____
W.E.T. SET   _____   _____
(10–20 min.)
_____   _____
_____   _____

Shake Out

_____   _____
_____   _____
_____   _____

Shake Out

_____   _____
_____   _____
_____   _____

Shake Out

Combination:_____   _____
_____   _____
_____   _____

COOL-DOWN   _____   _____
(5 min.)
_____   _____
_____   _____

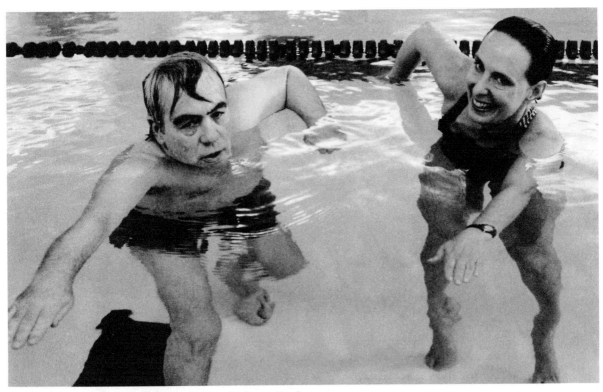

Author practices swim skills with famed columnist Jimmy Breslin.

W.E.T. Drills to Swim Skills

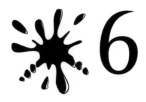

6

Basic Swim Skills with W.E.T.s

This chapter features W.E.T. drills for swim skills. Although it is not designed as a learn-to-swim program, this chapter presents a review of basic swim strokes which will be helpful for:

- ❑ the new swimmer
- ❑ the shallow water swimmer
- ❑ the "I used-to-swim" swimmer
- ❑ the "I-should-have-learned-to-swim" swimmer

The chapter highlights basic components of the standard swim strokes in addition to essential safety skills—floating and recovering to a vertical position. In addition, the all-important "breathing basics," for those who can swim but can't breathe properly, and need to master rhythmic breathing, are outlined. It helps you to transfer your W.E.T. exercises into fundamental swim techniques.

Each basic swim skill will be presented and illustrated. Then a sample W.E.T. drill will help you master this motion. In addition, boxed inserts give you further tips.

**W.E.T. TIP—
"Cornering Your
Partner"**

If you are swimming without a partner, use the corner of the pool for support and safety.

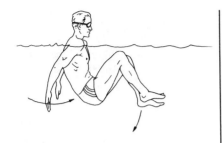

Back Float and Recovery

Becoming comfortable with the back float is the safety skill and is key to proceeding from non-swimmer to swimmer. However, many people may resist taking their feet off the bottom of the pool because they are anxious about getting their feet back on terra firma even while in the water. Therefore, it is helpful to simultaneously learn the back float *and* recovery to a standing position.

The Skill: Back Float and Recovery. Using a partner to support your head and shoulders, tilt your head, and lean back in the water until your feet rise off the pool bottom. Your legs, hips, and chest will rise toward the surface to a back float position. Your arms can either be at your sides or extended from the shoulders.

To recover to a stand, bend at the waist and simultaneously draw your knees up to your chest while you are lowering your chin. Scoop your arms behind you in a circular motion and lower your feet to the pool floor. (The motion is similar to that of seating yourself in a chair.)

W.E.T. Drill: Backward Jump Rope. Remember jumping rope? The backward jump rope movement helps to teach you this important safety skill.

Standing in waist- to chest-deep water, start with your hands behind your body. Bring your knees up to your chest as you bring your arms forward. As your arms pass your thighs, bring your feet back to the pool bottom; then pass your arms overhead, as in a reverse jump rope motion.

Breathing

Perhaps you've heard (or even said), "I can swim but I can't breathe." Most people hold their breath if their face is immersed in the water.

However, you should breathe similarly to how you breathe on land. And—*never hold your breath!*

The Skill: Breathing. Breathe regularly and continuously by inhaling out of the water through both nose and mouth, and exhaling under the water with nose and mouth as if whistling or blowing out through a straw. Review this breathing cycle by first standing in chest-deep water and breathe onto the palm of your hand, feeling the exhaled air flow.

W.E.T. Drill: Bobbing with Breathing. Practice breathing while bobbing at the pool wall. Inhale with face out of the water, and exhale with face submerged in water. This exercise not only accustoms the new swimmer to continuous inhalation and exhalation as the face enters and leaves the water, but it is also a good way of warming up and relaxing between W.E.T.s in a workout.

Face Float and Recovery

This skill helps you to become comfortable in the water in a prone (face in the water), streamlined position.

The Skill: Face Float and Recovery. Assume your overhead stretch position with your arms covering your ears, thumbs together, and bend forward from the waist. Inhale and at the same time bend your knees and push off from the bottom of the pool with the balls of your feet. As you lower your face into the water to forehead level, begin exhaling and straighten your legs behind you to assume a face float streamlined body position.

To recover to a stand, simultaneously bend knees, press arms downward at the sides, lift your head, and place both feet on the bottom. Practice the recovery to a stand first, by using the Forward Jump Rope W.E.T. drill.

W.E.T. Drill: Forward Jump Rope. Simulate jumping rope. As your arms bring the "rope" forward, bend your knees and lift legs to clear "rope." Continue jumping with your head lifting upward as "rope" arcs overhead.

Treading and Sculling

Treading is a safety skill that enables you to stay afloat in deep water in a vertical position, with your head above water, using as little energy a possible. To tread, your arms use a *sculling* motion and legs will kick in a bicycle *pedal action*. You can also use other leg kicks, e.g., scissor, eggbeater, frog, or whip kick.

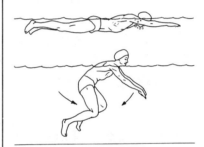

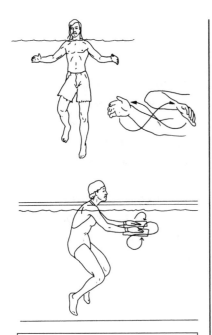

Sculling is a very important skill that also helps to improve your stroke efficiency. It is especially helpful in perfecting the "catch" of each armstroke. Sculling provides continuous support and propulsion.

The Skill: Treading Arm Scull Motion. Create a "figure 8" sculling motion by moving your arms simultaneously away from the center of your body and back to the starting point. Stand in chest-deep water with your arms extended in front of you just below the water's surface. Begin with thumbs up, palms facing each other. Turn your thumbs down and press your hands out and away from each outer until they are shoulder-width apart; then turn your thumbs up and press your hands toward each other until your palms almost touch.

Treading Bicycle Leg Motion. Move your legs in a bicycle pedaling action as if you were sitting on a bicycle seat, your shoulders hunched over your knees.

W.E.T. Drills: Paddle Scull and Marching Leg Steps.

Paddle Scull. In a vertical position, extend your arms forward, shoulder-width apart. With fingers pointed downward, create a "figure-eight" motion that moves your body headfirst. Use hand paddles as shown in the illustration. For added support, place a pull-buoy between your legs at your upper thighs.

Marching Leg Steps. Stand, then walk in shallow water, alternately bringing knees up toward chest as high as possible.

W.E.T. TIP

Practice Scull and Hug W.E.T. on page 27 and see sculling in chapter 9, "Synchronized Swimming." Use a flotation belt for extra support.

Strokes

Elementary Backstroke

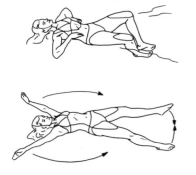

This stroke is relaxing and easy to coordinate because the body motions are simultaneous and symmetrical.

The Skill: Elementary Backstroke. Start in a back float position with your arms at your sides and your feet together. Your arms and legs move simultaneously. As you draw your hands up along the side of your body, bend your knees and lower your heels. When your arms extend into a V position, your heels will be extended approximately hip-width apart. Pull your arms straight down under the water to your sides while you snap your feet together. The sequence is "bend, extend, snap together, and glide." The combination is like the Aqua Jumping Jacks.

W.E.T. Drills: Scratch and Stretch Aqua Jumping Jacks.

Scratch and Stretch: Practice elementary backstroke arm motion in a standing position. Make believe you have an itch at your sides. Then stretch above shoulders in a straddle position. Pull straight down to sides and repeat.

Aqua Jumping Jacks. Start in chest-deep water with legs together and arms at your sides. Jump up, extending arms to the side. As you come down, your legs separate into a straddle position, your arms on the water's surface. Jump again, bringing arms down and feet together.

Crawl

The crawl stroke is usually the most popular stroke among Americans. Many people can swim crawl, but they have trouble mastering the breathing. The stroke uses an alternating flutter kick (like a walk) and an alternating hand-over-hand arm motion with stroke components of catch, pull, and recovery.

The secret to comfort while swimming the stroke is to get a steady supply of air. *Rhythmic breathing* is the coordinating of your arm strokes with your inhalation of air in a frequent, regular pattern.

The Skill: Crawl. As you turn your head to your breathing side to inhale, the arm of the opposite side of your body is stretched out in front of you. Take a breath and pivot your head into the water, exhaling and forming bubbles as that arm passes down and straight under your body. Remember to exhale continuously, never hold your breath, and pivot your head to the same side for your next breath.

This technique is *the* correct way to continuously maintain a breathing pattern while doing the crawl stroke.

W.E.T. TIP

Though the whip kick has superseded the "frog kick" for reasons of greater efficiency, many people find it to be an easier leg motion. In the frog kick, the knees bend outside hip width with feet close together and the legs extend into a wide V position before closing. Both the whip kick and the frog kick can be used for the elementary backstroke. Practice the Karate Kick W.E.T. drill on page 112.

SWIM TIP

Experiment with breathing on both sides to determine your better breathing side. Then practice your rhythmic breathing on that side *only*.

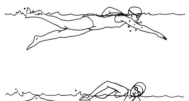

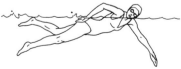

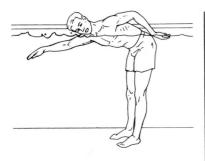

W.E.T. Drills: Breathe with Head Turn, Splashback, and Stroke and Breathe.

Breathe with Head Turn. Stand in waist-deep water, with your head in center position. Inhale as your head turns to your breathing side toward your right or left shoulder. Exhale continuously as your head turns back to center. Repeat to same side, maintaining continuous pivoting motion. Then, bend forward from your waist, place your face in the water, and practice the sequence of rhythmic breathing, forming bubbles continuously as you exhale.

Splashback: Walk in chest-deep water with the crawl arm stroke and splash water backward behind you forcefully as you finish the pull of each crawl arm stroke. You can also practice the splashback drill while holding a kickboard with one hand while splashing back with the other.

Stroke and Breathe: Combine the crawl arm motion and rhythmic breathing while standing in place.

W.E.T. TIP

Always keep your elbow higher than your hand throughout the arm motion. Practice with paddles.

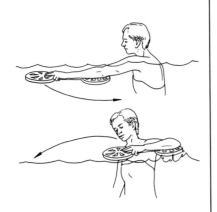

ELBOW LIFT STROKE CHECK

Starting Position: Stand in chest-deep water with arms extended in front of body, holding wand in each hand. Grasp handle of wand just under paddle; extend one or two fingers on top of paddle. The other paddle at the other end is just below elbow.

Technique: Practice crawl arm motion with paddle. Pull arm through water down to thighs, maintaining same posture. Then recover arm out of the water, barely clearing water with the wand and return arm to forward extended position. Repeat with other arm.

Backstroke

The other alternating stroke is the windmill backstroke. It is basically the crawl stroke done on your back; you breathe freely with your face out of the water.

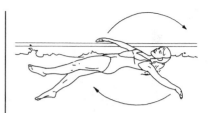

The Skill: Backstroke.
"Windmill" Arm Motion: Start in a streamlined backfloat position with arms at your sides. Lift one arm straight overhead while continuing to keep the other at your side. With pinky finger leading, press the overhead extended arm downward into the water for the *catch* of the windmill backstroke arm motion. Sweep this arm straight down under the water for the *pull*. Brush past your thigh with your thumb to complete the pull. *Recover* by lifting your arm out of the water, leading with your pinky to continue straight back to the catch position.

While the first arm is in midair recovering, the other arm is pulling. Continue the alternating arm stroke motion with arms moving continuously and in opposition to each other.

Flutter Leg Motion and Coordination. The backstroke flutter kick is similar to the crawl flutter kick. Your legs are close together and move in an alternating up and down motion. Your knees and ankles should stay loose. Kick water upward for maximum efficiency.

Alternating Backward Arm Circles. Alternately circle your arms backward, pulling under the water and recovering above the water. Make as large a backward circle as you can by raising your arm just past your ear and reaching as far back as you can.

Breaststroke

The breaststroke is a relaxing stroke done in face float position where the arms move in a heart-shaped motion simultaneously under water. The legs also move simultaneously underwater with a frog or whip kick.

The Skill: In a streamlined face float body position, trace the outline of an upside-down heart shape. For the *catch*, begin with your arms extended forward, thumbs pointing down. Press your arms outward and downward, palms leading for the *pull*. Bend

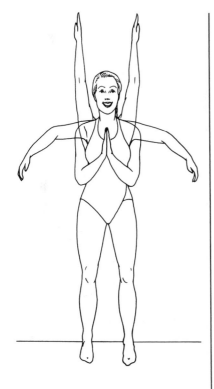

your elbows, keeping them up, and pull them back to shoulder level. Then bring your forearms together under your chest to complete the heart-shaped pattern. From this prayer-like position of hands and arms, *recover* underwater to the starting position by extending arms forward.

To breathe, your head lifts as you begin the arm stroke, and lowers with the recovery of your arm motion.

W.E.T. Drill: Heart-Shaped Pull with Breathing. Standing, then walking in chest-deep water, practice the heart-shaped arm motion as you breathe. Begin with your face in the water and your arms extended in front of you, thumbs touching. Lift your head to inhale as you begin to pull arms outward. As hands move under your chest, place your face back in the water and exhale, extending your arms in front of you.

W.E.T. Drill: Karate Kick. Stand in chin-deep water with your arms fully extended out away from your sides. Hold onto the pool edge for support. Keeping your knees close together, bend your knee and bring your right foot up behind you close to your right buttock. Then rotate your knee outward and touch the wall with your heel. Rotate your leg in a circle to resume the starting position. Repeat with the left leg.

Sidestroke

The sidestroke is a relaxing stroke which begins from a streamlined body position on either side that is done with your head just at the water's surface with your arms and legs remaining underwater.

The Skill: Sidestroke is a two-part stroke, beginning in a streamlined glide position on either side. In part one, both arms and legs move from a glide position to the midpoint of the body as you inhale. Part two is where both arms and legs meet in a tuck position and then extend and return to a streamlined glide position as you exhale.

The arm motion can be regular or overarm, while the leg-scissor kick can be regular or inverted.

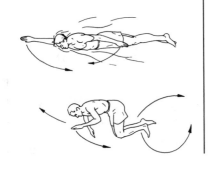

W.E.T. Drills: Apple Picking and Scissors Lunge.
Apple Picking: This drill simulates the sidestroke arm motion. Pactice by standing in chest-deep water. Extend one arm over-

head, reach, and "pick an apple from a tree." Place it in the other hand at chest level; then that hand throws it downward (as if into a basket). Reach for another "apple." Then bring your hands underwater, arms extended sideways. Practice "apple picking" with arms underwater in a standing position.

Scissors Lunge: Stand in chest-deep water with your feet together. Take a long lunge sideward with one leg bent at the knee, while your back leg remains straight. Draw your back leg up to meet the front leg as it straightens. Continue lunging forward; then change directions.

Butterfly

The butterfly stroke is perhaps the most exciting and is also perhaps the most energetic and challenging.

The Skill: The arms of the butterfly stroke move simultaneously recovering out of the water, tracing a "keyhole" formation. The dolphin kick is used where your legs move up and down,

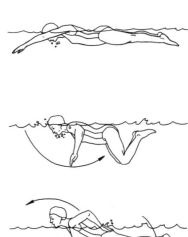

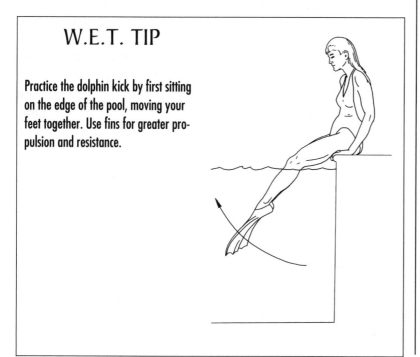

W.E.T. TIP

Practice the dolphin kick by first sitting on the edge of the pool, moving your feet together. Use fins for greater propulsion and resistance.

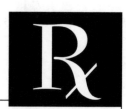

If you have any back concern, substitute other strokes for the butterfly in your W.E.T. swim workout.

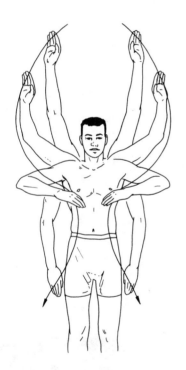

similar to the flutter kick, but in unison. A wave-like body motion is created by bringing your hips up (like a mermaid).

Butterfly Stroke with Single-Beat Kick: Although butterfly is normally done with a two-beat kick per arm stroke, the coordination of your arm and leg motion is best learned by starting with a single-beat kick per arm stroke. Begin in an extended face float position, arms extended overhead, hands shoulder-width apart for the *catch.* Bend your knees as you bend your arms for the *pull* and straighten your legs as you bring your arms above the water for the *recovery.* Lift your head for a breath as your shoulders rise during your pull.

W.E.T. Drills: Body Wave, Double Arm Circles, and Butterfly Lunge.

Body Wave: In deep water, hold on to the pool edge with one arm for support, keeping your body in a vertical position. With your legs together, press your hips alternately forward and backward, keeping your knees relaxed and allowing your hips and legs to move in a dolphinlike movement. To get the wavelike dolphin movement you can experiment using fins. You can also use fins to develop more propulsion, power, and flexibility. You're not cheating!

Double Arm Circles: Stand, then walk, practicing double arm circles with S-pull pattern. Brush your thumbs past your thighs before recovering arms out of water. This is similar to the jump-rope (page 106) arm motion.

Butterfly Lunge: Stand with your back against the pool wall, your arms extended to the sides, holding the edge. Place your feet on the wall, arching your back slightly. As you push off from the wall with your legs, lunge forward by recovering your arms over the water with the butterfly arm pull.

Crawl/Freestyle Swim Terminology

The terms "crawl" and "freestyle" are often used interchangeably. However, "freestyle" is sometimes the more efficient crawl stroke with additional refinements such as the S-shaped pull and body roll. The crawl/freestyle S-shaped pull is similar to the "keyhole" butterfly arm stroke. The right arm traces a reverse S pattern or question mark while the left arm traces an S pattern or reverse question mark.

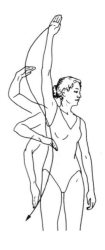

SAMPLE SWIM
W.E.T. WORKOUT

Comments:

WARM-UP
(5 min.)

_____   _____
_____   _____
_____   _____

W.E.T. SET   **Arm Motion:**
(10–30 min.)

_____   _____
_____   _____
_____   _____

Leg Motion:

_____   _____
_____   _____
_____   _____

Breathing:
  Bobbing with Breathing   _____
  Rhythmic Breathing   _____
  Crawl Arms and Breathe   _____

Coordination:
  Crawl and/or Back   _____
  Breast and/or Side   _____
  Medley of Strokes   _____

Optional: Lap Swim   _____
                                _____
                                _____

COOL-DOWN
(5 min.)
_____   _____
_____   _____
_____   _____

CREATE YOUR OWN SWIM
W.E.T. WORKOUT LOG

Comments:

WARM-UP
(5 min.)

_____   _____
_____   _____
_____   _____

W.E.T. SET
(20 min.)

Arm Motion:

_____   _____
_____   _____
_____   _____

Leg Motion:

_____   _____
_____   _____
_____

Breathing:

_____   _____
_____   _____
_____

Coordination:

_____   _____
_____   _____
_____

Optional: Lap Swim

_____   _____
_____   _____

COOL-DOWN
(5 min.)

_____   _____
_____   _____
_____   _____

LEARN TO SWIM
STROKE HIGHLIGHTS

STROKE	LEG MOTION	ARM MOTION	POWER FROM KICK	POWER FROM PULL
Elementary Backstroke	Whip Kick	Jumping Jack	50%	50%
Breaststroke	Whip Kick or Frog	Heart-Shaped	50%	50%
Crawl (Freestyle)	Flutter Kick	Alternating Straight Arm or S-pull	20%	80%
Windmill Backstroke	Flutter Kick	Alternating Arm Pull	25%	75%
Butterfly	Dolphin Kick	Keyhole	30%	70%
Sidestroke	Inverted or Regular Scissor	Overarm or Regular	50%	50%

Prescriptive W.E.T.s

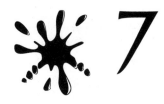

7

Water therapy has long been used for rehabilitating broken legs—of horses! Modern physical therapists have since learned to use water to help restore mobility and strength for people recovering from injuries and surgery, and for those with arthritis or other immobilizing conditions. The aim is to get them back into their daily home and work routines as soon as possible.

Recently, aquatic rehabilitation has moved beyond the traditional spa, to include the swimming pool as a rehabilitation medium. Use of a warm-water pool helps clinicians return injured athletes to participation in their chosen sport sooner than they would using only conventional land-based technique.

When an athlete is ready to return to active duty, usually at close to 100% of pre-injury strength levels, overall conditioning is again similar to that of the pre-injury state.

It appears that many sports-related injuries (leg, knee, ankle, hip, shoulder) can be rehabilitated in a shorter period of time using water exercise techniques as "water therapy" than with only previously used methods of dry-land rehabilitation.

Recently, therapists have been developing work conditioning exercises simulating job tasks to help prevent reinjury. This process begins with a reconditioning program, followed by a maintenance program.

Now you can use the buoyant and cushioning properties of water to relieve joint and muscle stiffness, and promote strength and flexibility in your own body. This chapter includes specific sample exercises to meet various physical situations.

The following are sample prescriptive strength W.E.T.s for strength.

GUIDELINES

Many aquatic facilities have a "family changing room" that accommodates those who need help getting suited up. These can be used by seniors, mixed-gender family groups that include young children, and those individuals who desire privacy while changing. This is a result of the guidelines recommended by the 1992 *Americans with Disabilities Act* (*ADA*), enacted to ensure that all facilities are accessible to all Americans. In addition to family changing rooms, many aquatic facilities offer stairsteps and ramps into the pool (which are easier to negotiate than vertical ladders), transfer chairs, and/or hydraulic pool lifts.

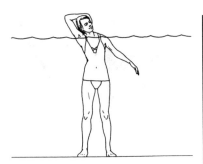

W.E.T. TIP

You can also do the warm-up Head Circles on page 23.

Strength W.E.T.s

LATERAL NECK FLEXION AND EXTENSION

Starting Position: Stand in neck-deep water with feet shoulder-width apart and arms extended to the sides.

Technique: Bring one hand over head and place on opposite ear. Keeping forearm parallel to water's surface, gently pull head toward shoulder. Release and stretch the other side.

FLEXIBILITY STRETCH

Starting Position: Stand in chest-deep water with arms extended overhead, and hands grasping kickboard at each end of its longest dimension.

Technique: This is a three-part, progressive flexibility stretch. From starting position, bend at the waist alternately from side to side. Then rotate the board lengthwise with hands

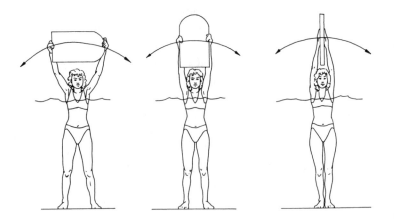

grasping the width of the board, keeping arms overhead and straight, and repeat movement from side to side. Complete the flexibility stretch by holding the board at its narrowest width, with palms pressed inward and arms still straight overhead.

Equipment: Kickboard.

ARM AND SHOULDER DECK STRETCH

Starting Position: Stand in chest-deep water near pool wall, with one arm extended straight and grasping edge of the pool.

Technique: Rotate body, decreasing its angle to the wall so that your shoulder is gradually and progressively stretched. Place your other arm on the wall and stretch your opposite shoulder.

Variation: Place back against pool wall, with hands holding onto wall or gutter and arms extended beyond shoulder width. Slowly "walk" hands closer to shoulder width, stepping forward slightly. Bring hands as close as possible to each other. For an extra challenge, slowly lower body by bending knees to chin level.

HORIZONTAL WATER WALK

Starting Position: Float on your back in the corner of the pool, grasp edges for support.

Technique: Turn onto your side and practice a walking motion; then turn onto your other side to move in the opposite direction.

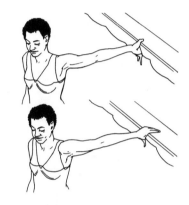

W.E.T. TIP

Practice this exercise with your thumb first upward, then downward, so that you engage both biceps and triceps (antagonistic) muscle groups.

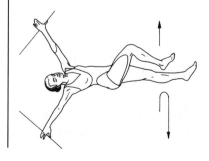

W.E.T. TIP

Practice helicopter W.E.T., page 76.

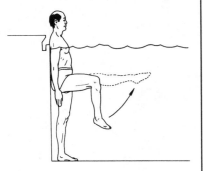

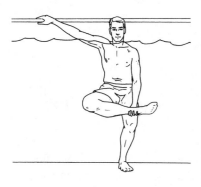

W.E.T. TIP

If this exercise brings relief to your feet, also try Runner's Calf Stretch.

KNEE LIFT

Starting Position: Stand with back or side against pool wall, paying attention to good posture.

Technique: Bend knee, bringing thigh parallel to water's surface. Extend leg forward at knee; then bend it and return leg to pool bottom, while standing leg remains slightly bent. Repeat on other side.

HIP FLEXOR

Starting Position: Stand in waist- to chest-deep water, with back resting against pool wall for support.

Technique: Cross one leg in front of body, grasping ankle. Gently hold ankle, stretching muscles at hip and back of thigh by bending the standing leg. Then return to standing position. Release and change to other side.

SHIN CURLS

Starting Position: Stand in waist- to shoulder-deep water, holding onto pool wall for support.

Technique: Raise one foot and slide it slowly up and down the shin of the other leg. Try to grab the shin with your toes. Return foot to floor and repeat with the other foot.

CALF STRETCH

Starting Position: In waist- to chest-deep water, face pool wall and lean forearms on edge. Place feet shoulder-width apart, with toes on the wall and heels on bottom, with toes pointed outward.

Technique: Slowly bring chest and abdomen toward the wall, creating a calf stretch.

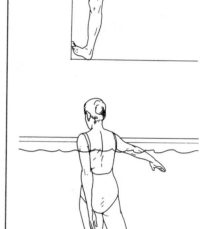

ALTERNATE TOE TOUCH

Starting Position: Stand in chest-deep water with arms extended to the side, and pay attention to good posture.

Technique: Raise heel to buttock, and reach behind body to touch heel or ankle with opposite hand. Return foot to pool bottom and repeat on opposite side. Keep bent knee pointed to the pool bottom.

Activities of Daily Living

Basic strength training exercises have been cited as a means of retaining and even restoring independent living for seniors or anyone else who is becoming less active. The buoyant properties of water make aquatic exercise ideal for those who are convalescing from long illness or surgery, or for anyone who is severely deconditioned. While some of these exercises may seem very basic, it has been found that movements that were previously difficult on land can be performed more easily in a pool or spa, because of buoyancy. These same movements can be transferred back to land, making everyday activities easier.

Having a relative or companion assist some exercisers during their water exercise workout and in the locker room will make these sessions safe, enjoyable, and productive.

1. Walking—preserve and improve mobility by walking in the water, focusing on good posture. Travel in different directions (forward, backward, sideways) and with different steps: grapevine (hora dance step), braiding, etc. Then walk with knees brought as high as possible toward chest.

2. Climbing stairs—practice moving up and down stairs using an aquatic step. Place step close to pool wall for support and balance if needed.

3. Reaching for door and turning knob—Reach forward below water's surface with alternate arms. Close fist and rotate palms upward. Bend elbow and bring arms back toward body, and beyond. Exercise can be combined with an aqua step and can be done with web gloves.

4. Key turns—Small motor movements to keep fingers strong and limber: "turn" keys or knobs underwater, open and close fists, "play" musical instruments, flex fingers, grasp small objects. Other things to practice are writing your name, dialing important phone numbers, touch-tone dialing (and the TV remote!), turning the pages of a newspaper or book, buttoning or unbuttoning, eating with fork, knife, or spoon.

5. Balance for walking—Holding a kickboard at water's surface with each arm. The water will help support you and there is less danger of falling. Or bring an aluminum cane into the pool and practice walking.

6. Rising from chair:

a) Upper body: To regain biceps/triceps strength, stand in midriff- to waist-deep water with knees hip-width apart and slightly bent, so that forearms are on water's surface, parallel to pool floor, with palms down. Press hands down while straightening knees. Then bend knees again, bring hands up to surface with thumbs facing upward. For support, exercise near wall, with back leaning on wall.

b) Lower body: Holding onto edge of the pool for support, lift leg forward to strengthen abdominal muscles. Turn around and repeat on other side, raising opposite leg. Or in water that is at least chest-deep, place back against the wall and hold onto pool edge for support. Lift both legs together with knees bent, knees together if possible. Then return them to pool bottom. Try with legs straight.

7. Putting on a coat, blouse or shirt—In chest-deep water, pass a kickboard from left to right, back to front. Practice putting on slacks or a skirt by lifting one leg at a time as high as possible, holding pool edge or flotation device for support. Then bring one or both hands to alternately raised foot for socks or stockings.

8. Cooking—To increase strength and agility for kitchen activities, stand in chest-deep water with arms under the water's surface. Cross (but don't fold) arms in front of body. Rotate forearms forward, then backward around each other. Then reach arms forward alternately, adding a grasping motion with your hands (to pick up a pot or dish, or open a cabinet, etc.) and then bring them back to crossed position.

9. For general upper arm strengthening—In chest-deep water, do a Trunk Twist, keeping elbows as high as possible, ideally at water's surface.

10. Use water jets—massage afflicted area with warm water from jets of the spa.

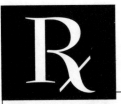

There are many different types of arthritis. The most common are rheumatoid arthritis and osteoarthritis, which, although they have different symptoms, can both be relieved by water exercise. Speak to your physician about exercising in the water; get information on what type of exercises will be most beneficial for you.

W.E.T. TIP

See Arm and Wrist Swirls on page 24, which may also be helpful to enhance your range of motion.

Arthritis W.E.T.s

The aim of using W.E.T.s for the arthritis patient is to increase mobility and develop small motor movement during the water workout, and then transfer the increased flexibility back to land. Greater range of motion in the water will provide comfort as well as greater mobility out of the water. Some arthritis sufferers say that their return to an independent lifestyle is partly due to the result of water exercise.

Many exercises in *The New W.E.T. Workout* may be used for an arthritis water workout. The following exercises are fundamental to restoring and maintaining range of motion in important joints. Exercises in warm water (approximately 84° to 86°) will be most comfortable, and may relieve pain and stiffness.

HAND AND FOOT SMALL MOTOR MOVEMENTS

Starting Position: Stand in waist- to shoulder-deep water near pool edge, with hands and arms underwater.

Technique: Begin with the smallest movements of opening and closing fingers from each other, then

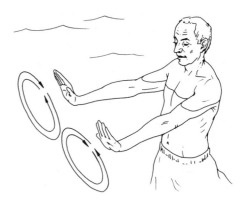

opening and closing your fist. Then from a neutral position (hands open, as if palms are resting on a table), point your fingers upward, then downward (flexion and extension), and then inward and outward (lateral movement). Then combine these movements into a circular movement in each direction, with fists open or closed.

For foot movement, hold onto pool edge for support as needed. Raise one foot slightly from the pool floor, rotate ankle several times to the left, then the right. Return foot to pool floor and rotate the other ankle, as comfort allows.

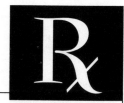

Be sure to work at your comfort level. If you experience pain during your workout, decrease the intensity of the exercise or stop exercising.

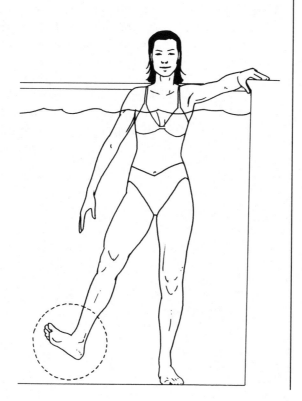

FIGURE-EIGHT MOVEMENTS

Starting Position: Stand in waist- to shoulder-deep water near pool edge, with hands and arms underwater.

Technique: Starting from a neutral position (hands open, as if palms are resting on a table), with elbows close to body, perform figure-eight sculling motion.

For foot movement, hold onto pool edge for support. Raise one foot in front of body, and describe a figure-eight with your foot, first to the right, then to the left. Return foot to pool floor and repeat on the other side.

Variation: For an energetic variation, draw a large figure-eight with each leg. Start with one foot in front of your body, swing leg in close to the inside of your other foot and then back out behind your body, as far as comfort allows. Then bring your leg back under your body and swing it forward, extended in front of the body to the starting position.

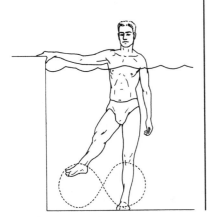

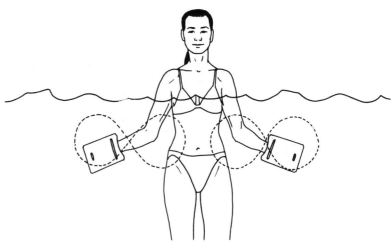

Mastectomy W.E.T.

- ❑ Often there can be stiffness in the area of the surgery, as well as numbness. It can also be harder to raise an arm. Water helps with flexibility, which needs to be worked on continually.
- ❑ Edema is a common problem for mastectomy patients. The hydrostatic pressure of the water helps to remove fluids, helping to reduce stiffness.
- ❑ Stretching the arms above the head may be a problem. Practice elementary backstroke, at first with arms out to the sides. Progressively bring arms past shoulder level.
- ❑ Some women find abdominal exercises more difficult. Swimming or kicking on a kickboard will gradually increase flexibility.

MASTECTOMY EXERCISE

Starting Position: Stand in chest-deep water with elbow near waist and forearm out to the side.

Technique: Move arms towards, then past, the midline of the body and up to the water's surface.

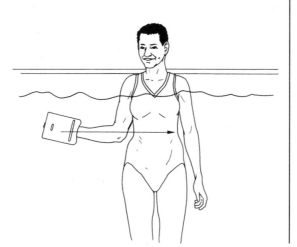

"Fifteen years ago, six weeks after my daughter was born, I had a mastectomy. Not knowing how to swim at the time, I never imagined we would do laps together when she got older. After year of watching her swim classes, I became inspired. When I found out that there was a special inexpensive prosthesis for bathing suits, I became hopeful.

Now I swim and water-jog regularly, and there is an added benefit that I did not anticipate. Exercising in the pool is a sure way of cooling my menopausal hot flashes."

Associate Prof. Laura Greenberg
Dept. of Art, Music and Philosophy
City University of New York
John Jay College

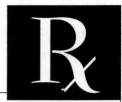

Ask your doctor about other water exercises.

HYDROTHERAPY

Hydrotherapy refers to the use of water to accelerate healing or relief. This includes water in all its forms: solid—ice; liquid—water; gas—steam. Hydrotherapy includes moving water: home whirlpool baths, Swedish "needle" showers, or the traditional "Hubbard tank" often used in hospitals for treatment of injuries.

Father Sebastian Kneipp, a nineteenth-century German priest, was a founder of modern-day hydrotherapy. He used cold Bavarian rivers to transform himself from an unwell teenager to a strong and vigorous adult. The Kneipp spa in Germany continues to use the hydrotherapy and herbal treatments he developed.

Hydrotherapy is used to bring relief to both muscles and ligaments (connective tissue). Sports-medicine specialists use head and ice alternately to attend to injuries, and physicians prescribe water exercise to relieve chronic conditions.

CRYOTHERAPY

Ice therapy, also known as cryotherapy, is the therapy of choice for reducing tissue swelling, decreasing a given pain, relaxing and increasing circulation to affected part.

The use of ice to treat an injury goes back hundreds of years. Today, injured people will often run to the refrigerator to get ice. Makeshift ice packs can even consist of boxes of frozen food wrapped in a towel. In addition, gel packs can be stored in the freezer for emergencies, and can be reused. New technology has developed substances that become cold after impact; these do not need cold storage, but are only for one-time use.

The application of cold reduces swelling in order to decrease internal tissue pressure, thus reducing the amount of fluids outside the injured tissues. This allows blood to circulate more freely. Cold also causes internal

---

ICE TIP

A ready-to-use ice compress can be kept on hand by freezing water in a small paper cup. Store in freezer; when needed, peel off the top of the cup (like peeling an orange), cover the ice with cloth or a paper towel, and apply it to the injury. Continue to peel away cup as the ice melts.

biochemical changes to help healing in tissue, in addition to reducing pain by causing numbness.

The most recent trends recommend that, generally, ice be applied to an injury for 20 minutes, followed by one hourwithout cold to let tissues return to normal, and then ice again for 20 minutes, and again one hour off. After the third ice application, wait 5 to 6 hours before repeating the process. A faster, but probably less efficient method, is to apply ice for 10 minutes, off for 20 minutes, and so on. Ice can be used from immediately after an injury through 3 to 4 days or even more after the trauma, as opposed to the 72 hours previously recommended.

Ice can also be used where there is no visible swelling, to open blood channels. This is often used as a preventive measure for athletes participating in vigorous sports. Though the athlete is unable to see internal swelling, it is presumed to be present.

HEAT

Heat increases blood circulation. Warm applications cause internal tissue not too far below the skin to bring in more blood, which increases oxygenation of the affected area and promotes the carrying away of waste products such as lactic acid, reducing pain. The warmth itself is a pain reducer because sensory nerve endings interpret the warmth both to the brain or spinal cord as a relaxant—it feels good.

Heat treatment is often in the form of a compress, a towel soaked in hot tap water (sometimes including herbs such as eucalyptus) which is then wrung out and firmly wrapped around the affected area, but not cutting off circulation. Other modalities include mud, salt, and paraffin.

Spas are useful for treating sprains; epsom or other salts in the spa sometimes offer relief for neuritis, muscle fatigue, and arthritis.

Generalized applications of heat such as steam baths (wet heat) and saunas (dry heat) are cleansing agents for non-traumatic situations. The heat causes the body to perspire, which increases blood circulation and is relaxing.

Moist-heat therapy is excellent for increasing local and/or peripheral blood circulation. It also acts as a relaxing agent.

Morton Steuer, D.C., M.S.
Doctor of Chiropractic Medicine
U.S. Modern Pentathlon Team

RELAXATION FLOAT

Starting Position: Stand in waist- to chest-deep water, wearing flotation equipment.

Technique: Lean backwards, letting feet float off the pool bottom, until you are in the back float position. Use floating position to take pressure off back, neck, legs, or feet.

Equipment: Flotation belt, buoyancy collar or W.E.T. vest, ankle floats, wrist floats.

Variation: While floating, extend arms overhead. Try doing the Triceps Stretch (page 19) with both arms underwater.

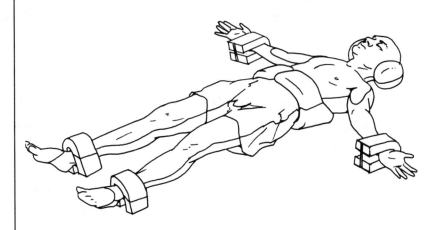

CREATE YOUR OWN PRESCRIPTIVE W.E.T. WORKOUT

W.E.T. WORKOUT LOG

Comments:

WARM-UP
(5 min.)

_____   _____
_____   _____
_____   _____

W.E.T. SET
(10–30 min.)

Upper: _____   _____
_____   _____
_____   _____

Shake Out

Middle: _____   _____
_____   _____
_____   _____

Shake Out

Lower: _____   _____
_____   _____
_____   _____

Shake Out

Total: _____   _____
_____   _____
_____   _____

COOL-DOWN
(5 min.)

_____   _____
_____   _____

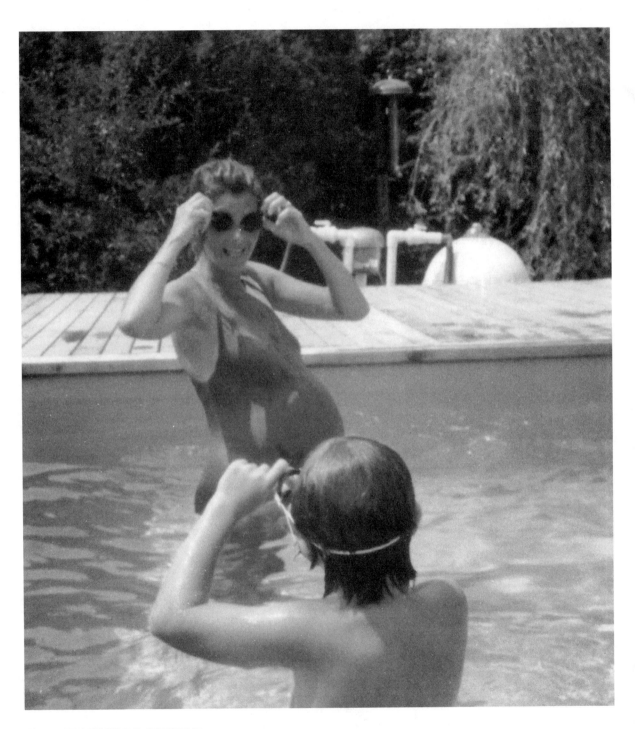

Pregnancy W.E.T.s

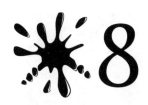

8

If you are pregnant, planning to be pregnant, exercise with women who are pregnant, or know someone who is, then this chapter is for you.

Most obstetricians encourage their patients to engage in some form of physical conditioning because they believe that a woman who is in good physical condition may be less likely to have difficulty during her labor and childbirth. Even women who were not physically active before pregnancy now are encouraged to start exercising.

The first chapter of *The New W.E.T. Workout*® highlights the benefits of exercise: strong heart and lungs, good circulation, and optimum oxygen utilization. A healthy system is all the more important during pregnancy because the mother's blood supply will increase 25% to 50% during pregnancy. Blood must be efficiently transported from the mother's body to the placenta, which provides the baby with oxygen and nourishment. A sensible fitness program will enable the heart to handle this and other demands with greater ease.

For the pregnant woman, exercising in water has definite advantages. It minimizes the stress, strain, and pounding that often accompanies land exercise. It helps many women control their weight during pregnancy. A mother-to-be ideally gains from 20 to 30 pounds during a normal pregnancy; water exercise can help keep off extra pounds. And water is soothing and relaxing.

Since the uterus is surrounded by abdominal and pelvic floor muscles that help to support it, good abdominal muscle tone is helpful during pregnancy. Strong back muscles also help to accommodate the growing uterus, lessening the stress on the back, hips, and thighs. A good fitness program should help the

The known benefits of exercising during pregnancy refute the ideas held in previous generations that exercise would harm a woman's reproductive organs, and that exercise during pregnancy is dangerous to the unborn child. The uterus is a very well-protected organ, guarded by strong ligaments and surrounded by pelvic bone. The unborn child is well protected from injury by the abdominal wall and the strong uterine muscle as well as by the amniotic fluid and sac.

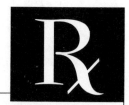

A pregnant woman should not begin an aquatic fitness or any other exercise program without the knowledge and approval of her doctor.

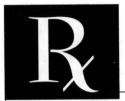

Do not use a spa if you are pregnant, or think you are. The fetus does not have an "air conditioning" system; overheating can cause problems.

pregnant woman to strengthen abdomen, back, and shoulder muscles to help carry the weight more easily and maintain good posture, which is so important for a comfortable pregnancy. And water exercise may help minimize postpartum difficulties as well.

A water exercise program during pregnancy can also be used to prepare muscles and joints for childbirth itself. A mother who is in good condition is better prepared for the physical demands of labor and delivery.

Water exercise can increase cardiovascular efficiency. This advantage is a plus in handling the additional demands that pregnancy places on the heart and circulatory system, and can also reduce blood pressure. Improved cardiac efficiency may help to minimize swelling (edema) in the extremities, as well as help avoid varicose veins. And just being in the water has a diuretic and nutriuretic effect; that is, it causes the body to naturally rid itself of excess water and salt, which are often causes of edema and discomfort as well as the much-to-be-avoided high blood pressure. This many also reduce the stiffness, caused by water retention, that some pregnant women experience at the ankles and wrists.

The support provided by the water itself facilitates blood flow and helps to relieve the pressure exerted on the bladder and pelvic organs. And, being horizontal keeps the exerciser off her feet, which not only feels better but reduces the likelihood of varicose veins. Finally, improved fitness helps minimize the fatigue most women experience during pregnancy.

POSTURE CHECK

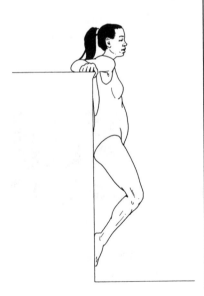

Starting Position: Stand in chest-deep water with feet together and soft knees, with your shoulders, back, buttocks, and heels against the pool wall. Grasp the pool edge with both hands for support. The small of your back should be against the wall.

Technique: Bend your knees and place your feet flat against the pool wall, supporting yourself.

Keep your arms straight. Breathe regularly. Hold for a count of 10, then rest.

Variation: You can also practice a variation of this exercise at home. Lie on the floor with your knees bent and your feet flat on the floor, as close to your buttocks as possible. Lift your hips off the floor, so that your body is straight form your knees to your chest. Inhale through your nose as you lift your hips and exhale through your mouth as you lower your legs.

PELVIC TILT

Starting Position: Stand in waist-deep water with your back and hips against the pool wall. Place your feet as close together as possible. Rest your arms on the pool ledge for support.

Technique: Tilt your pelvis upward by pressing the small of your back toward the wall, while turning your face downward. Hold the tilt for a moment, then slowly relax back to the starting position. Breathe normally.

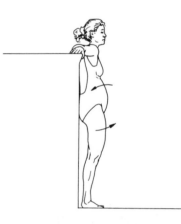

CALF STRETCH (LADDER/STAIR)

Starting Position: In waist-deep water, stand with legs together on a pool step or a ladder rung. Place your weight on the balls of your feet so that your heels project over the edge. Hold onto the stair or ladder railing for support.

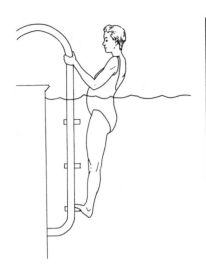

Technique: Stand on tiptoes; then lower your heels until they are below the rung or step. Return to tiptoes and repeat. Breathe regularly.

Variation: If you do not have a safe, comfortable ladder available for your workout, face the pool wall, standing arm's length away. Grasp the edge, step forward with one foot, and shift your weight onto your forward leg, keeping your feet flat on the pool floor. In this lunge position, you will feel the gentle stretch in the calf of your back leg. Then reverse your legs. Try to keep your back leg straight. If the stretch pulls too much, bend your back knee slightly. Keep practicing until your muscles are loosened.

SWING AND SWAY

Starting Position: Face the pool wall and hold the edge with both hands shoulder-width apart and arms extended. Place your feet together on the pool floor.

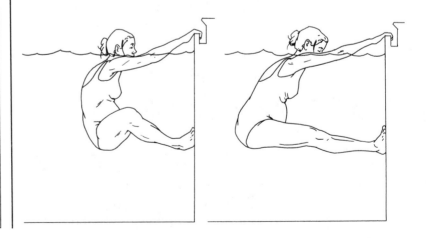

Technique: Bending at the waist, walk up the wall with knees bent and apart until your feet are at hip level. Then straighten your knees, bringing your body away from the wall for a count of five. Flex your knees a few times, bringing your body slowly near and away from the wall. Then swing your hips from side to side, feeling the stretch in your buttocks and upper legs. Breathe regularly.

EFFLEURAGE

Starting Position: Stand in the pool at any comfortable water depth or float on your back.

Technique: Place your fingers on your navel, pointed slightly downward. Trace a circular design on your abdomen with your fingertips in a continuous motion for approximately one minute.

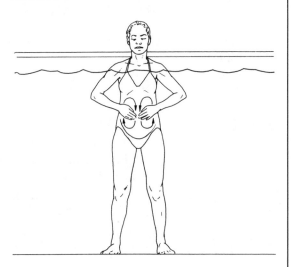

W.E.T. TIP

In the Lamaze method, effleurage becomes a conditioned reaction to any tightness in the abdomen as pregnancy progresses. You can also use effleurage between exercises and with different breathing patterns.

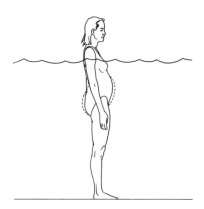

W.E.T. TIP

Try the Shoulder Shrug in conjunction with the massage. With your arms relaxed at your sides, roll your shoulders backward, then forward several times. Then lift and roll each shoulder separately. (See p. 23.)

You can also use the Shoulder Shrug instead of the Back Massage if you are exercising without a partner.

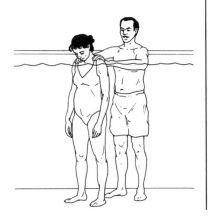

WATER KEGEL

Equipment	Flotation support (optional).
Starting Position:	Stand in chest-deep water with your feet less than hip-width apart.
Technique:	Tighten your lower abdominal muscles, then contract your pelvic floor and vaginal muscles. Release your muscles. After 10 repetitions, hold the contraction and your breath for five to 10 seconds; then release and exhale.

You can repeat the sequence several times during your workout.

You can also use a flotation support to allow your feet to float off the pool bottom.

BACK MASSAGE

Starting Position:	Stand in shoulder-deep water, feet comfortably spaced, with your childbirth coach standing behind you.
Technique:	Have your partner gently massage your back beneath the surface of the water.

Have your partner use the heels of the palms. Relax and breathe regularly. The back massage combined with the soothing properties of the water will make you feel wonderful!

Sample Pregnancy W.E.T. Workout

Warm-Ups

Water Walking

Aqua Lunge

Cross Chest Stretch

Posture Check

Main Set

Water Push

Sit-Ups

Aqua-Jog

Kickboard Presses

Circle Spray

Back Extension

Knee Lift

Calf Stretch (Ladder/Stair)

Swing and Sway

Leg Swirl

Cool-Downs

Pelvic Tilt

Water Kegel

Effleurage

Back Massage—with partner (optional)

W.E.T. TIPS

❑ Strong back and abdominal muscles may help minimize lower back discomfort as pregnancy progresses.

❑ Exercises that help stretch the inner thigh can be helpful during labor and delivery.

LEGEND

WU	=	warm-up
LB	=	lower body
MB	=	middle body
UB	=	upper body
TB	=	total body
CD	=	cool-down

Pregnancy Exercises

WU	Pelvic Tilt
WU	Water Kegel
LB	Swing and Sway
LB	Calf Stretch (Ladder/Stair)
CD	Back Massage—partner exercise
CD	Effleurage
CD	Posture Check

W.E.T.s in Other Parts of Book— Useful During Pregnancy

WU	Bobbing with Breathing
WU	Aqua Lunge
WU	Standing Tall
WU	Cross Chest Stretch
WU/TB	Aqua-Jog
UB	Kickboard Presses
UB	Push-Ups
UB	Water Push
UB	Sculling
MB	Circle Spray
MB	Trunk Twist
MB	Sit-Ups
MB	Back Extension
MB	Knee Lift
LB	Wall Walk
LB	Ballet Leg Stretch
LB/WU	Runner's Calf Stretch
TB	Treading
TB	Water Walking

GENERAL PREGNANCY WORKOUT TIPS

The American College of Obstetricians and Gynecologists (ACOG) has developed guidelines for exercise safety during pregnancy and the postpartum period. Here are highlights of the ACOG recommendations that pertain to water fitness.

PREGNANCY AND POSTPARTUM

1. Regular exercise (at least three times weekly) is preferable to intermittent activity.
2. Avoid vigorous exercise in hot, humid weather or when your are running a fever.
3. Avoid ballistic (jerky or bouncy) movements.
4. Precede vigorous exercise with a five-minute warm-up period. Follow vigorous exercise with a period of gradually declining activity that includes gentle stationary stretching.
5. Measure heart rate at times of peak activity and avoid exceeding target heart rates and limits established in consultation with your physician.
6. Drink liquids liberally before and after exercise to prevent dehydration. If necessary, interrupt activity to replenish fluids.
7. If you have a sedentary lifestyle, begin with low-intensity physical activity and advance levels gradually.
8. Stop activity and consult your physician if any unusual symptoms appear.

PREGNANCY ONLY

1. Limit maternal heart rate to not more than 140 beats per minute.
2. Limit strenuous activities to 15 minutes in duration.
3. Don't exercise in the supine position after the fourth month of gestation.
4. Make sure caloric intake is adequate to meet not only the extra energy needs of pregnancy, but also of the exercise performed.

These guidelines were originally published in 1985. Since then, new information about the responses of a pregnant woman and her baby to exercise has become available. Women who began pregnancy already fit and participating in vigorous activity felt that the original guidelines were too conservative. The new findings indicate the following:

1. Women who had been exercising previous to becoming pregnant were better able to respond to heat or cold.
2. Fetal breathing and body movements increased during exercise, indicating fetal well-being.
3. Most babies born to women who exercised were within a normal range of birth weights.

CREATE YOUR OWN
PREGNANCY W.E.T. WORKOUT

Comments:

WARM-UP
(5 min.)

_____ _____
_____ _____
_____ _____

W.E.T. SET   **Upper:**_____ _____
(10–30 min.)
                        _____ _____
                        _____ _____

                        Shake Out

                        Middle: _____ _____
                        _____ _____
                        _____ _____

                        Shake Out

                        Lower: _____ _____
                        _____ _____
                        _____ _____

                        Shake Out

                        Total: _____ _____
                        _____ _____
                        _____ _____

COOL-DOWN   _____ _____
(5 min.)
                        _____ _____
                        _____ _____

Synchronized Swimming W.E.T.s

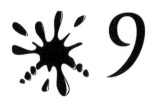

9

Water ballet, the sport of synchronized swimming, is rhythmically performed swimming synchronized to music. In Europe, where it began, it was originally known as "ornamental swimming." This aquatic activity is often compared to figure skating because both combine the aesthetic concerns of an art form with the rigors of sport. Synchronized swimming is an Olympic sport. It has come a long way since Esther Williams.

Body positions and figures, combined with stroke variations, sculling, and treading, give synchronized swimming its grace and visual balance. With consistent training, synchronized swimming greatly increases stamina and breath regulation; the entire body is toned and strengthened, especially the shoulder, leg, and abdominal muscles.

If you're a regular water exerciser, or have decided to become one, the inclusion of this graceful and creative activity in your workout will make your swim more fun, more interesting, more challenging, and a better all-around exercise. Some of the exercises can be done in the corner of a pool, while others can be incorporated into lap swims. Synchro exercises offer a wide range of moves to stretch and condition every part of you.

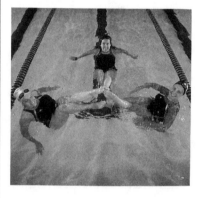

Basic Skills

The sculling arm motion is perhaps one of the most important ways to practice with hand paddles. There are several exercises;

Is "synchro," as it is nicknamed, a sport or an art? It is both. As a sport, it requires rigorous training, endurance, strength, breath control, and responsive muscle coordination. In addition, the swimmer learns to synchronize movement to music by counting beats. The art is in making the choreography seem effortless and graceful.

one is with sculling and hand paddles. It is hard to describe and much easier to feel with hand paddles on. This can be done for a treading motion, which is also an excellent way to perfect that figure-eight motion.

Components of Synchronized Swimming

Sculling

The main arm component in synchronized swimming is sculling. There are many sculling variations. The basic one for propulsion and support is *headfirst sculling*, in which the hands and forearms following a figure-eight pattern (the infinity sign), pushing water toward the feet with the body moving head first. In a back float position, the hands are at the sides, close to and behind the hips, with fingertips pointed upward.

Sculling uses the same basic figure-eight motion as in stationary treading. Sculling allows you to move in different directions, and it supports your body in different positions. Five water ballet exercises that you can incorporate into your post-turn program follow. See page 30 to review the basic sculling motion.

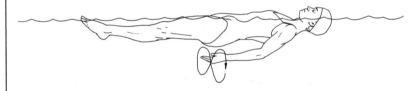

Tips for Effective Sculling

As with any new activity, build up your sculling strength and endurance slowly. Start with just a lap (up to 25 yards) at a time of each movement described above, and gradually increase the

Torpedo sculling: Extend your arms behind your head and flex your wrists backward so that your fingers point outward and your palms face away from your body throughout the scull. You will move toward your feet. Torpedo sculling will help you develop a streamlined body position.

distance (or time, with vertical sculling) as you become stronger and more proficient.

Give your hands and forearms a break if they start to feel tired or sore during a sculling workout by adding some gentle flutter kicking. If your muscles start to cramp, stop sculling. Stretch and massage the area; then gradually resume sculling.

Scull vigorously to develop hand, arm, and shoulder strength and endurance; scull gently to ease into a workout or cooldown.

Since the S-pull used in your freestyle stroke is really a big scull, you can improve your stroke technique by slowing down and analyzing your sculling movements. You'll find that this helps develop a better "feel" for the water.

Be courteous when sculling in the pool. Use the slow lap lane, keep an eye out for those in front and behind you, and allow swimmers to overtake you at the wall.

Treading

Treading is the other component of synchronized swimming; it combines a sculling arm motion and one of a number of leg motions. It provides support and movement in the water.

The most common form of treading uses the bicycle pedal kick to help push the body upward (see page 108 of chapter 6). Synchronized swimming also uses treading with a scissors or frog kick.

Another kick, which is very energetic, is the "egg beater," where the legs circle inward one after the other (see Karate Kick W.E.T. drill, page 112).

Tug-of-War

The Tug-of-War on page 48 is a combination W.E.T. The arms use a reverse or support scull, and the legs use a treading motion. As the arm motion pushes the body downward, the leg treading holds the body up on the water. You can have a tug of war with yourself by doing this exercise. Synchronized swimmers often train with hand paddles or swim mitts to develop their vertical sculling skill.

EQUIPMENT TIP

Various swim toys can enhance your sculling practice. Hand paddles (full or half) help strengthen your wrists and forearms, while swim mitts and webbed gloves increase the power of your scull. You may also want to use a pull-buoy for lower body support, and fins for lower-body propulsion.

SUPPORT SCULLING

Have you seen synchronized swimmers upside down with their legs high in the air? No, they are not touching the bottom of the pool but are doing support sculling. Here the swimmers' arms sweep like windshield wipers, moving outward from, then inward to the center of the body. The elbows are kept close to the waist and the palms are flat, facing the surface of the water. To develop support sculling skills, practice the Tug-of-War exercise.

Body Positions

Synchronized swimming uses several body positions. A sequence or series of movements within a position is called a figure. Following are basic body positions and an example of a figure for each.

Back Layout

Begin on back in back-float position with face, hips, thighs, and feet close to the water's surface, toes pointed, with the body streamlined and hands sculling close to hips.

TUCK TURN

Starting Position: Begin in the back layout position.

Technique   Bring your knees toward your chest, keeping shins close to the water's surface.
    Remaining in the tuck position, turn your body 360°, pushing the water by turning your palms sideways in the opposite direction, keeping your face above the water. Repeat, going the other way.

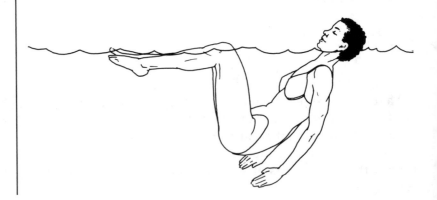

CLAM

Starting Position: Begin in a back layout position.

Technique: With your arms, create a downward and overhead circular movement as the hips pike, drawing your straightened legs to your chest. Move your hands out of the water to approach your feet before submerging.

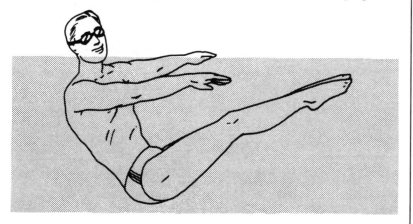

MARLIN TURN

Starting Position: Begin in a back float (layout) position with your arms extended at shoulder level. Your face, hips, thighs, and feet are at the water's surface.

Technique: Roll your body to the right one quarter of a turn as your legs move a quarter turn to the left on the surface. Use your arms to move the legs and body out to face a new direction. Make a total of four quarter turns (90° each) as close as possible to the surface of the water. Repeat in the opposite direction.

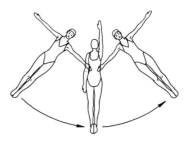

BENT-KNEE MARCHING STEP

Starting Position: Begin in the back layout position with hands sculling at hips.

Technique: Lift and bend one leg so that your thigh is perpendicular to the water's surface.

Continue to scull faster just under your hips. Straighten leg and repeat on the other side.

Variation: If you are having difficulty keeping the straight leg on the surface, place it on the pool's edge or have someone support you lightly under your ankle.

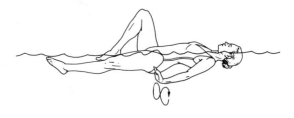

SHARK CIRCLE

Starting Position: Begin in a back layout position. Turn to either side to assume a side layout position with body arched. The top arm is extended overhead, close to the water's surface, next to your ear.

Technique: Scull with your lower arm to move your body in a complete circle on the surface.

Complete your Shark Circle by resuming your back layout position.

Variation: Reverse direction.

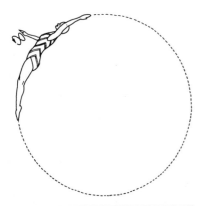

SWIM STROKE VARIATIONS FOR SYNCHRONIZED SWIMMING

Stroke	Head	Arm Motion	Leg Movement
Crawl	Head remains forward and out of water	Straight-arm recovery	Bent-knee flutter kick underwater
Breaststroke	Head remains out of water. Turn head at the catch after each stroke	Hands splash on recovery	Flutter kick underwater
Backstroke	Chin up; head remains still	Windmill backstroke or salute stroke	Slow bent-knee flutter kick underwater
Sidestroke	Head remains still or alternates moving forward and back	Alternate overarm with regular arm pull	Alternate scissors with flutter kicks on glide

Sample Workout

Let there be music! You can practice your movements to poolside music, or even listen to music with a waterproof tape player or radio. Experiment with different types, tempos, and moods to create your own set of movements in a water routine.

Synchronized swimming can be an addition to or an extension of your W.E.T. workouts. For example, you can combine these swim stroke variations in different ways to create your own routine.

- Alternate the crawl and backstroke every three strokes.
- Alternate the sidestroke with the breaststroke, changing sides.
- Combine all the strokes while moving in the same direction—breaststroke, one sidestroke, one backstroke, one crawl stroke, breaststroke.
- Create your own combinations.

Sample Synchro W.E.T. Workout

Warm-Ups (5 min.)

Water Walking

Treading

Main Set (20–30 min.)

Includes: sculling, figures, strokes, and combinations. Rest when needed.

Sculling and Leg Motions

Scull 50 yards, head first (fingers upward) in back layout position.

Karate Kick

Figures

Bent-Knee Marching Step

Clam

Marlin Turn

Shark Circle

Tuck Turn

Strokes—Medley of Strokes

Swim 25 yards using the crawl stroke and the backstroke.

Swim 25 yards using the breaststroke and the backstroke.

Swim 25 yards creating your own stroke variations.

Cool-Down (5 min.)

Cross Chest Stretch

Aqua Lunge

Arm Stretch

CREATE YOUR OWN
SYNCHRO W.E.T. WORKOUT

Comments:

WARM-UP
(5 min.)

_____   _____
_____   _____
_____   _____

W.E.T. SET
(20–30 min.)

Sculling:_____   _____
_____   _____
_____   _____

Shake Out

Figures:_____   _____
_____   _____
_____   _____

Shake Out

Strokes: _____   _____
_____   _____
_____   _____

Shake Out

Combinations: _____   _____
_____   _____
_____   _____

COOL-DOWN
(5 min.)

_____   _____
_____   _____
_____   _____

W.E.T. Variations and Other Water Environments

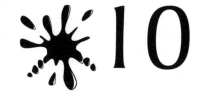

Spa W.E.T.s

Along with regular swimming pools, many health clubs and Ys offer water amenities known variously as whirlpools, spas, and hot tubs.

The following spa stretches are designed to help relax the body. These exercises can be used for general well-being, as well as to help certain ailments such as arthritis, fatigue tensions, and/or limited range of motion. They are isometric or static in nature (two forces pressing against each other). Your total spa time should be no longer than 15 minutes. Use the jets for intensified water-massaging action on various body parts such as ankle, knee, shoulder and wrist joints, and back.

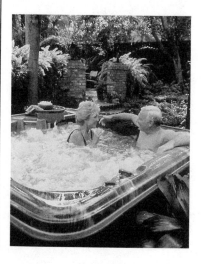

FOOTSIES

Starting Position: Sit on the edge of the spa with your feet just at the water's surface.

Technique: Rotate the lower legs so that your feet turn:
- ❑ inward
- ❑ outward
- ❑ forward and backward (up and down)
- ❑ sideways

Variation: Mix and match your foot circles as you're sitting on the edge of the spa

SPA SIT 'N' KICK

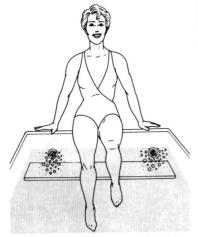

Starting Position: Sit at the edge of the whirlpool

Technique: Begin with a slow rhythmic flutter kick—alternate kicks, e.g., dolphin (loose), breast-stroke (flex feet as much as possible), etc. Concentrate on kicking slowly and try to keep your ankles flexible.

Variation: Change the intensity and speed of the kicks: 30 seconds of each kicking; 30 seconds of rest; 30 seconds of moderate kicking; 30 seconds of rest.

SPA SIT 'N' STRETCH

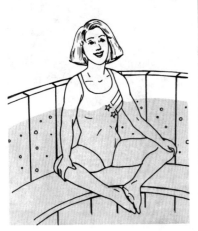

Starting Position: Sit in the bent-knee position, soles of the feet together.

Technique: Press your knees toward the bottom, stretching the inner thigh.

Variation: Rock from side to side.

V VICTORY STRETCH

Starting Position: Sit in the corner of the tub with your back against the wall and your legs in a V position, the knees straight.

Technique: Separate your legs as far as possible, trying to touch the wall with your legs in the V position. Keep your legs straight and bring them together slowly, alternately crossing one leg over the other.

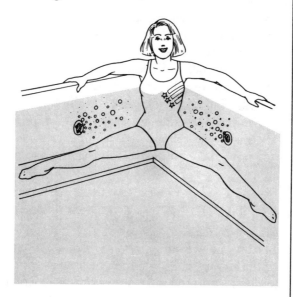

CROSS LEG STRETCH

Starting Position: Sit in spa with one leg flat on spa bottom while the other leg crosses it at the knee.

Technique: Grasp your lower leg, and slowly pull thigh upward toward your chest, stretching thigh area (adductors and abductors) of crossed leg. Change legs and repeat on the other side.

Spa Safety Checklist

1. Check with your doctor before using a spa, especially if you have heart disease, hypertension, diabetes, kidney disease, or chronic skin problems.
2. If you are pregnant, avoid using the spa. The fetus has no "air-conditioning" system of its own, and serious problems could result from overheating.
3. Don't use the hot tub alone; in the event of an emergency, someone should be present.
4. Don't wear jewelry in the spa; the metal can become uncomfortably hot.
5. Do not do vigorous exercise in the spa.
6. Don't drink alcohol before using the spa; it may increase your risk of heat injury.
7. Remember to hydrate; water is the best.
8. Do not use the spa immediately after vigorous exercise; this also increases your risk of fainting.
9. Limit your time in the spa to 15 minutes.
10. Enjoy the relaxing environment of a spa—acrylic materials now make atttactive home spas affordable for many people.

Pool W.E.T.s

Fixtures in swimming pools which are a part of the construction of the facility can sometimes be used as water exercise equipment and incorporated into your workout. Here are some samples:

DANCER'S LEG STRETCH

Starting Position: Stand in chest-deep water facing ladder or other pool structure, grasping both rails of ladder.

Technique: Place one leg onto ladder step and extend other leg behind body. Keep that foot flat near pool bottom, stretching hamstrings.

Try to keep hips level to each other. Return forward foot to pool bottom and bring other leg forward to ladder step.

Variation: Begin on a low ladder step, and as your flexibility increases, place forward foot on a higher ladder rung.

LATERAL LADDER STRETCH

Starting Position: Float on back, holding onto ladder or other pool structure.

Technique: Straighten legs and stretch out from ladder. Then move from side to side by bending your arms alternately, and swinging your body in the direction of the bent arm.

Open Water and Beach W.E.T.s

Water, Water Everywhere . . . Open-Water and Beach Activities

The following are suggested W.E.T.s for an outdoor, open-water environment.

Sand Jog

Jog in calf-deep water at the beach. The deeper the water, the more energetic.

W.E.T. TIPS

- ❑ Be certain that pool or lane space is available to do this without interfering with others.
- ❑ Use the pool entry steps (at the shallow end of many pools) as an aquatic step. Strengthen your lower body by stepping up and stepping down, holding onto handrail for support.
- ❑ Aqua shoes are recommended.

SAFETY TIP

When outdoors, remember to apply waterproof sun protection: sunglasses, hat/visor.

Crabwalk

Sitting at the water's edge, place your hands next to your hips. "Walk" forward, backward, and sideways, allowing legs to drag. For variation, do the Crabwalk in the push-up position. The more your body is in the water, the easier it will be.

Sandy Sit-Ups

At the water's edge, bury your feet in the sand, bend your knees, sit up, and touch one of your elbows to the opposite knee. Repeat with the other elbow.

Fins, Mask, and Snorkel

In open water, fins can be used to aid in movement through the water; a snorkel enables you to breathe with your face in the water; and a mask provides underwater vision, covering both nose and eyes.

If you have a neck problem, and are not able to use rhythmic breathing, you will be able to swin continuously with a face mask and snorkel.

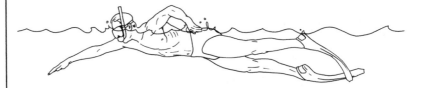

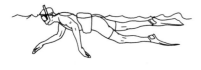

If you have a shoulder problem, swim in a prone position using a "dog paddle" motion, keeping your hands under the water. Use a flotation device to help you remain at the surface.

Surfer's Arm Stroke

From a balanced prone (face down) position on a raft or surf board, propel yourself using alternating forward arm circles (crawl stroke) or (simultaneously) a butterfly stroke.

Family W.E.T.s

The following are examples of water activities which can be done with your family members. Introducing your little one to the water can be a good exercise, and it can be a great deal of fun, too.

Play "motorboat" or train engineer—here, you're going to pull your little one through the water and encourage him/her to kick and just let him/her enjoy the water, and always maintain eye contact with your child.

To help your child go underwater, pretend it is his/her birthday and the cake is waterproof and it is under the water. Have him/her "blow out" (exhale) all of the candles under the water.

For the family with four or more people, play a version of Ring Around the Rosy. Here, you can practice submerging and going down to form bubbles. If there are a lot of people in the pool, play a "ball game" such as water polo, water volleyball, water basketball (try a water hoop), or a simple game of catch with a light beach ball. These games are fun for both youngsters and for the young at heart. These games will get everyone going by involving everyone.

ABC W.E.T.s

Starting Position: Stand in waist- to shoulder-deep water. Hold onto wall or flotation device for support if needed.

Technique: Outline letters or numbers with feet, e.g., the alphabet, your name, your shopping list, social security number, waist size, etc.

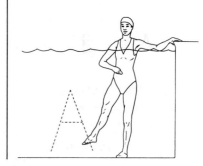

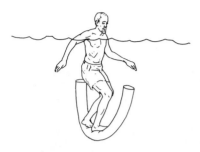

LOG RACE

Starting Position: In deep water, away from wall obstructions and other people, grasp log in the middle, and submerge it under body. Place one foot in front of hand. Still holding the log, place second foot behind first foot. Release hand from log and slowly find equilibrium on log.

Technique: Use sculling motion to propel body forward or backward, bending or straightening knees according to comfort and to maintain optimum balance.

Equipment: Log (½ or full length)
Optional—mitts for sculling

Variation: Stand on log width-wise for easier balance.

KICKBOARD SIT

Starting Position: Standing in water that is at least chest deep.

Technique: Place a kickboard behind you using both hands, and assume a sitting position. Use your arm movements for both balance and locomotion.

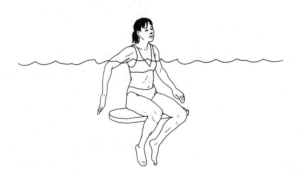

PORPOISE DIVE

Starting Position: Stand in waist- to chest-deep water, facing the pool.

Technique: With a plyometric (bounding) motion, jump off the bottom of the pool, clearing the water's surface, and then glide underwater as far as possible.

W.E.T. TIP

Be careful in shallow pool not to dive too deeply.

Partner W.E.T.s

Some W.E.T.s can be done by two people. Have a good time with a "water buddy" by doing these effective strengthening and stretching exercises together.

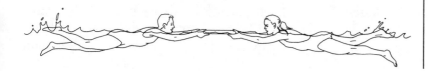

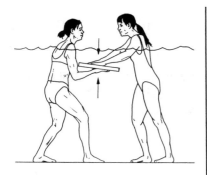

KICKBOARD PRESS

Starting Position: Partners stand facing each other in waist- or chest-deep water with a kickboard held width-wise between them at the water's surface.

Technique: One partner presses up on the kickboard while the other presses down at the same time. This provides an isometric effect.

KICKBOARD RACE

Starting Position: Each partner holds a kickboard lengthwise in front on their body, with arms extended, either standing in the water or at the pool wall.

Technique: Partners use the kick of any stroke to cross the pool (e.g., flutter kick), competing for speed, according to agreed-upon guidelines. (See Competition W.E.T.s, page 167.)

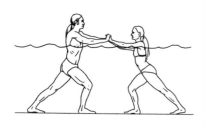

PARTNER HAMSTRING STRETCH

Starting Position: Partners stand in waist- to chest-deep water, facing each other, with arms extended forward, and pressing palms together (left to right, right to left) with equal pressure.

Technique: Each partner bends right knee and places right foot in front of his/her body, with left leg extended behind the body. Heels remain on pool bottom. Each partner leans forward, exerting equal pressure for approximately 15–30 seconds to stretch hamstring and calf muscles. Then reverse the stretch by placing left knee forward.

PARTNER QUADRICEPS STRETCH

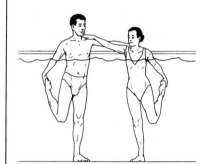

Starting Position: Partners stand in waist- to chest-deep water, supporting each other at the shoulders.

Technique: With their outside hands, each partner leans forward, keeps the knees together, and grasps their own outside foot, bringing it as close to the buttocks as possible. Hold the stretch for 15–30 seconds, then break hands, turn around, and stretch the other leg.

DOUBLE WATER WHEEL

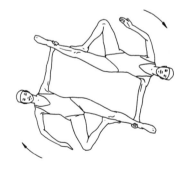

Starting Position: Partners float side by side in back layout position in opposite directions (head to toe, toe to head). Each partner bends the right knee, with right instep against the inside of the left knee.

Technique: Each person holds partner by left ankle with his/her hand. Using the right hand for figure-eight sculling, and keeping it close to your hip, move "wheel" around in a circle in the direction of the bent knee.

At-Home W.E.T.s

Home-Sweet-Home Water Activities

In your own bathtub do static arm and leg stretches; shoulder shrugs; breathing; buttock squeezes; and foot, ankle, and wrist circles. Try Sit 'n' Stretch in the bathtub.

Isometric exercises can also be done in a tub. An isometric exercise is a contraction of the muscles in which the length of the muscle does not change. Here, you'll use your muscles to push or pull against an immovable object—the bathtub wall.

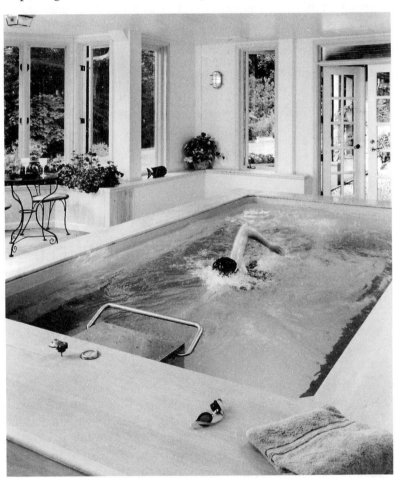

Press your hands against the inside of the tub wall in a sitting position. Hold for a maximum of 30 seconds and relax. Here your breath is held during your isometric exercise. Breathe deeply between contractions.

Depending on the size of your tub, try an isometric leg press with your feet pressing against the front of the tub. Hold for a maximum of 30 seconds and relax.

Competition W.E.T.s

In classes, intramural events, summer clubs, and recreational outings there are a variety of fun and competitive W.E.T. games and events in which everybody—including adults, teens, and children—can participate. Games which can be played in the pool are:

- ❏ volleyball
- ❏ basketball
- ❏ soccer
- ❏ shallow water polo
- ❏ water Frisbee

or relay races can be set up with two or more groups competing. Here are some ideas:

Water Walking/Running Races: Events at distances from 1 width to 500 yards (e.g., 25 yards, 50 yards, 100 yards, 200 yards). Also, they can be set up as an "Individual Medley" of strokes. These can be done moving forward and/or backward.

Participants should wear aqua shoes.

Water Exercise Techniques routine:
A sample five-minute routine including:
    1 minute warm-up
    3 minute main set (upper, middle, and lower body exercises)
    1 minute cool-down

Add appropriate musical accompaniment.

TRIATHLON CHALLENGE

One of the most exciting competitive events yet devised is the triathlon, where swimming, running and cycling are combined in various distances. They can begin at small distances and range ultimately to the Ironman Triathlon, which features a 2.4 mile swim, 106 mile bike ride, and a 26.2 mile run! That's a full day's work. However, variations exist (thankfully); a mini-triathlon could be made up of a 10 minute swim, a 10 minute stationary bike ride, and a 10 minute treadmill run, all tracked for distance. The swim here could even be a water walk, if you don't swim *yet*. Of course, there will always be those for whom a triathlon is steam, shower, and sauna. . . .

Deep Water Running Races: From 25 yards to 200 yards. Contestants should wear flotation belts.

Relays: Combination of teams such as two coed teams; up to 8 individuals can compete.

COMPETITION FIN SWIMMING

Fin swimming as a competitive sport, using regular bi-fins or monofin, is gaining in popularity. The Underwater Society of America (USOA) sponsors an annual U.S. National Fin Swimming Championship meet.

Fin swimming competition is divided into three categories for both men and women.

1. *Surface Competition Events*—usually swum freestyle with fins added. Distances range from 100 yards/meters to 1,500 yards/meters.
2. *The Apnea Event*—a breath-holding sprint of 50 yards/meters swum entirely underwater. The use of the monofin has dramatically advanced the sport of fin swimming with the current men's apnea record at 15.4 seconds for a 50-meter sprint!
3. *The Immersion Event*—swum in distances of 100 to 400 meters with a small scuba tank. They are open only to those with scuba certificates.

CREATE YOUR OWN W.E.T. WORKOUT
(FOR OTHER WATER ENVIRONMENTS)

Comments:

WARM-UP
(5 min.)

_____   _____
_____   _____
_____   _____

W.E.T. SET   **Upper:**_____   _____
(10–30 min.)
                        _____   _____
                        _____   _____

Shake Out

Middle: _____   _____

                        _____   _____
                        _____   _____

Shake Out

Lower:_____   _____

                        _____   _____
                        _____   _____

Shake Out

Total:_____   _____

                        _____   _____
                        _____   _____

COOL-DOWN   _____   _____
(5 min.)
                        _____   _____
                        _____   _____

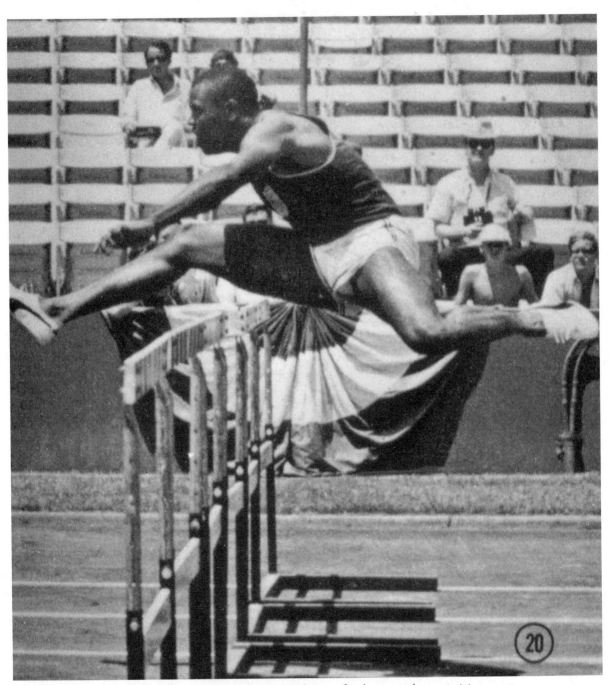

Five-time Olympian Willie Davenport uses Water Exercise Techniques for therapy and cross training.

Qs and As for Your W.E.T.s

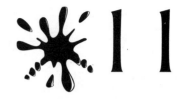

Getting Started and Keeping at It

Q. *Am I too old to start an exercise program?*

A. You're never too old to start an exercise program. However, if you have not been physically active, I strongly urge you to get a physical examination and a stress test, especially if you're over 35. If your physician says you're in good shape to begin an exercise program, then by all means get started. Generally speaking, water exercise is probably the best all-around activity for somebody who is starting out on the road to physical fitness. Certainly it is not as strenuous or bone-jarring as jogging. Many over-40s are out there exercising, and they are doing amazing things; so age should not be a barrier to starting a program of physical fitness.

Remember the unique benefits of water: buoyancy (you perceive your body weight to be approximately 10% of your body weight on land), relaxation, increased range of motion, improved cardiovascular system—and most of all, it's refreshing and fun!

Q. *Will I experience any discomfort doing W.E.T.s?*

A. You should feel that you have had a rewarding workout; however, if you experience any serious discomfort during your workout, stop and rest, then continue. If the discomfort continues, your body is trying to tell you that something is

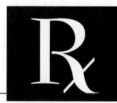

Remember to check with your physician before starting this or any exercise program.

not right, and you must stop and see your doctor. Always listen to your body.

Q. *My muscles are too tight; will I be able to use W.E.T.s?*
A. Yes, but start with the relaxed version of the exercises. As you progress, your muscles will become more supple and the exercises will become easier for you.

Q. *Why do I feel stiff and sore after a W.E.T. workout, and what can I do about it?*
A. You may experience some discomfort at the start of your W.E.T. program because you're using muscles that have been inactive. Be certain to warm up properly. You may wish to switch to the relaxed versions of specific W.E.T.s. If pain or discomfort persists, consult your doctor.

Q. *Why do I get cramps and what can I do about them?*
A. A cramp is a contraction, or tightening, of muscle fibers. It is usually caused by lack of a warm-up or by overexertion. There is a warning sign; you feel tension in the area, usually the leg. This should be your signal to stop or ease up. Listen to your body.

    If a cramp does occur, apply direct pressure to the area by squeezing and pressing the affected muscle deeply with your thumbs. Rest before continuing your W.E.T.s.

Q. *What should I do when I feel discouraged about my progress?*
A. Don't give up. The road to physical fitness is never short, and it requires dedication and self-discipline to reach your goals. So when you hit the doldrums, just remind yourself that at the end of the road there will be a healthier and happier you. Hang in there and go for it!

Q. *I'm so busy during the week that I really don't have the time to exercise—I can only exercise on the weekends. What can I do about this?*
A. Get your long exercise sessions in on the weekends, and try to supplement these with shorter sessions during the week—try to exercise at least twice during the week. Remember that there are 24 hours in each day, and after sleep and

work, you should have at least eight hours left. Schedule one hour for exercise—no matter what, you should try to get that one hour for yourself. Discuss this with your family, associates, and friends; if they see you are determined to get fit, I am sure they will support your efforts—and who knows, you may involve some of them.

Q. *How much time should I devote to a W.E.T. routine?*
Ideally, do your W.E.T.s three times per week. Begin with a 20-minute workout, including a five-minute warm-up, a 10-minute W.E.T. set, and a 5-minute cool-down.

Q. *Why do I feel tired after exercising?*
A. Your aerobic capacity is developing and improving, and if you have not been exercising regularly, you may feel tired. Start with the relaxed variation of W.E.T.s and try to follow the program for at least three times a week. Exercising regularly will ultimately give you more energy. Stay with it!

Q. *Can I do W.E.T. workouts during my menstrual period?*
A. There is no reason why you should not. If you experience discomfort, you may be more comfortable doing the "relaxed" level of your W.E.T.s.

Balancing Diet and W.E.T.s

Q. *If I go on a weight reducing diet, why do I have to exercise?*
A. Dieting alone may help you lose excess weight, but diet and exercise together will help you reach your ideal weight much more quickly. Also, dieting alone will not firm up your muscles and improve your shape; only exercise can do that. Many dieters are disappointed because they frequently regain their lost weight, but a consistent exercise program can help break that cycle and keep you at your ideal weight.

CALORIC BURN

Caloric burn is most accurately determined by the oxygen consumption level of the muscles. However, your heart rate is more easily used as a reference for your workout intensity. Recent research indicates that walking 3 miles per hour can burn up to 500 calories in thigh high water, and that the amount of calories burned during water walking increases with the depth of the water. A half hour of deep-water running burns about 300 calories, compared with about 200 to 250 for land running, 150 for playing tennis, and 150 to 200 for aerobics.

When swimming, a 150-pound person swimming at his target heart rate (THR) burns approximately 10 calories a minute, which is approximately 600 calories per hour.

Q. *As long as I am exercising, do I have to worry about my diet?*
A. Exercise alone will not use up enough calories to help you lose weight unless you are going to exercise for two to three hours a day—which, for most of us, is not possible. Diet and exercise should always go hand in hand.

Q. *How many calories should I consume to lose weight or maintain a desired weight?*
A. This depends on several factors—age, activity level, health, individual metabolism, etc. However, if you're over 21, approximate your required caloric intake by multiplying your desired weight by 15. For example, if you want to maintain a body weight of 120 pounds, your daily caloric intake would be about 1,800 calories (120 x 15 = 1,800). Keep in mind that if you are physically active, your daily caloric intake should not drop below 1,200. Remember that exercise and dieting go hand in hand in weight reduction.

Q. *How can I calculate weight loss?*
A. There are 3,500 calories per pound of body weight. If you eat 500 fewer calories a day and maintain the same activity level, you would start to lose weight. If you used up 3,500 calories per week your net weight loss for the year would be about 50 pounds. After your W.E.T.s your metabolism is increased, which helps to burn more calories.

Q. *If I exercise, should I increase my intake of protein?*
A. Not necessarily. Your body uses carbohydrates for its fuel, and you should eat more of these, but in the form of fresh fruits and vegetables, grains, and grain products. Be sure you eat a balanced diet that provides you with the required vitamins and minerals. Try to drink at least eight glasses of water a day to replace the water you lose through perspiration.

Q. *I've heard that exercise acts as an appetite suppressant. How does it do this?*
A. As you exercise, the blood that is not needed in your stomach and intestines is shunted to your heart, lungs, and muscles

where it is needed. Research has shown that after your exercise session, it may take up to three or four hours for the blood to return to your stomach. Until that time, your body cannot digest food very well; therefore, you often do not feel the need to eat. This is your body's way of telling you to wait before you eat.

The Food Pyramid

The food pyramid of the U.S. Department of Agriculture (USDA) was developed to provide guidelines for good nutrition for the general population. (Consult a health-care professional if a special health condition, such as diabetes, exists.)

The basic objective of the pyramid is to encourage you to eat a *variety* of foods. No one food, no matter how wholesome it is, can provide all the nutrients needed for good health. With this in mind, you should choose foods from the six food groups in the pyramid each day and vary the foods in each group from day to day.

In order to present the true nutritional content of foods without the confusing language of advertising hype, the standard Nutritional Facts label was developed. The box on the right side of the label gives guidelines for the typical daily percentage values of essential nutrients needed for good health. The list below it gives the ingredients in the products in descending order. The panel on the left of the label gives the number of grams, and the percentage, of the recommended daily value (based on a 2,000-calorie diet) of the essential nutrients listed on the right side of the panel. The gram is a unit of weight (28.4 grams equals one ounce), and the calorie is a unit of energy.

Applying this to the two labels shown side by side for a whole apple and for a typical slice of apple pie, it is easy to see that choosing the apple allows you to stay more readily within the guidelines.

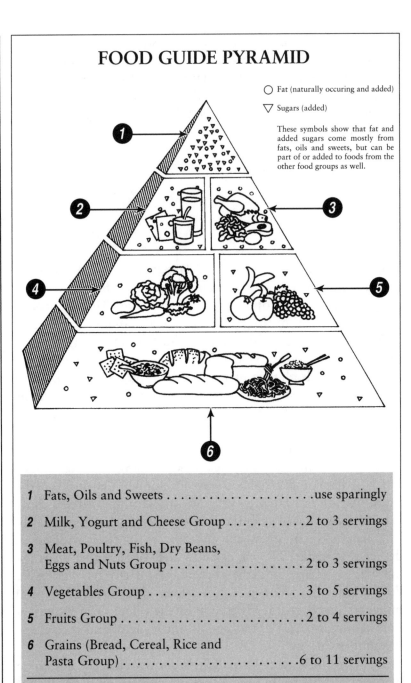

FOOD GUIDE PYRAMID

○ Fat (naturally occuring and added)

▽ Sugars (added)

These symbols show that fat and added sugars come mostly from fats, oils and sweets, but can be part of or added to foods from the other food groups as well.

1 Fats, Oils and Sweets . . . . .use sparingly

2 Milk, Yogurt and Cheese Group . . . . .2 to 3 servings

3 Meat, Poultry, Fish, Dry Beans, Eggs and Nuts Group . . . . .2 to 3 servings

4 Vegetables Group . . . . .3 to 5 servings

5 Fruits Group . . . . .2 to 4 servings

6 Grains (Bread, Cereal, Rice and Pasta Group) . . . . .6 to 11 servings

The U.S.D.A./D.H.H.S. food pyramid illustrates the food groups and the amounts of food that should be consumed from different groups.

Nutrition Facts

Serving Size Medium size Apple
Servings Per Container One (180 mg)

Amount Per Serving

Calories 96	**Calories from Fat** 0

	% Daily Value*
Total Fat 1g	1.5%
Saturated Fat 0g	0%
Cholesterol 0g	0%
Sodium 7mg	0%
Total Carbohydrates 24g	8%
Dietary Fiber 2g	8%
Sugars 15g	
Protein 0.3g	

Vitamin A 4%	•	Vitamin C 12%
Calcium 1.5%	•	Iron 3%

* Percent Daily Values are based on a 2,000 calorie diet. Your daily values may be higher or lower depending on your calorie needs.

	Calories	2,000	2,500
Total Fat	Less than	65g	80g
Sat. Fat	Less than	20g	25g
Cholesterol	Less than	300mg	300mg
Sodium	Less than	2,400mg	2,400mg
Total Carbohydrates		300g	375mg
Dietary Fiber		25g	30g

Calories per gram
Fat 9 • Carbohydrate 4 • Protein 4

INGREDIENTS: Apple

Whole (fresh) apple

Nutrition Facts

Serving Size Medium 1/6 of 9-inch Pie
Servings Per Container Six

Amount Per Serving

Calories 410	**Calories from Fat** 152

	% Daily Value*
Total Fat 18g	28%
Saturated Fat 5g	25%
Cholesterol 6g	2%
Sodium 480mg	20%
Total Carbohydrates 60g	20%
Dietary Fiber 1g	4%
Sugars 20g	
Protein 3.4g	

Vitamin A 1%	•	Vitamin C 3%
Calcium 0%	•	Iron 3%

* Percent Daily Values are based on a 2,000 calorie diet. Your daily values may be higher or lower depending on your calorie needs.

	Calories	2,000	2,500
Total Fat	Less than	65g	80g
Sat. Fat	Less than	20g	25g
Cholesterol	Less than	300mg	300mg
Sodium	Less than	2,400mg	2,400mg
Total Carbohydrates		300g	375mg
Dietary Fiber		25g	30g

Calories per gram
Fat 9 • Carbohydrate 4 • Protein 4

INGREDIENTS: Apple, water, enriched wheat flour, sugar, vegetable shortening, corn starch, butter, salt, vanilla, spices, baking soda

"Typical" apple pie

You're Beautiful with W.E.T.s

Q. *What kind of bathing suit is best for doing my W.E.T. workouts?*

A. Choose a bathing suit that is comfortable, lightweight, and becoming to your body. Be certain that there are no uncomfortable string or strap placements that can rise up or slip down and that your buttocks and bust are secure. Lycra is comfortable, and one size does fit most people; however, check the life of your suit if you use it often—Lycra suits will eventually develop threadbare areas at the hips, bust, or buttocks. The life of a nylon suit is longer, but many people find them less comfortable. There are also various combination fabrics available on the market. Whatever your suit is made of, be sure to rinse it thoroughly after each use to prolong its life.

Q. *Is chlorine harmful?*

A. Chlorine is used in pools to keep them free of bacteria and algae. It won't hurt you. However, the combination of chlorine and water can dry your skin and hair. There are state-of-the-art water treatments that eliminate the use of chlorine.

Q. *What can I do to protect my skin?*

A. Use your favorite moisturizer just after your W.E.T. workout. Shower as usual, and apply your moisturizer to moist skin to help replace the natural oils that have been depleted by the water.

Q. *Can I protect my skin from the sun's rays while doing my W.E.T. workouts at the beach?*

A. Yes, use a waterproof sunscreen with PABA and a high sun protection factor. After your W.E.T. workout, reapply the sunscreen because it will wear off after a period of time because of perspiration and water.

Q. *What can I do to protect my hair?*

A. If you need to keep your hair dry, choose W.E.T. workouts that keep your chin above water. Also use a sweatband

According to the Center for Disease Control, there are no known cases of HIV/AIDS contracted in a swimming pool.

around your hairline to help protect it against any surprise splashes. You can protect your hair with a bathing cap, too. For extra protection, apply your favorite conditioner to your hair ends. Remember to shower after each W.E.T. workout, and apply a hair conditioner or creme rinse.

Q. *Should I wear goggles while doing my W.E.T. workouts?*
A. Most of your W.E.T. workouts can be done without submerging your face. However, if you wear contact lenses and/or you are combining your W.E.T. workouts with swimming, goggles are recommended. (Prescription goggles are available.)

Q. *How can I protect my ears during W.E.T. workouts?*
A. Many of the W.E.T.s are done with your head above water. If you wish to prevent water from entering the ear canal, I suggest the following:
   ❑ *Ear plugs:* These seal your outer ear canal; they are reasonably priced and easily available.
   ❑ *Lamb's wool:* (available in drugstores and swim stores) Place a small piece of lamb's wool in your outer ear canal and seal it with petroleum jelly.
   ❑ *Bathing cap:* Use a snug-fitting bathing cap that covers your ears.

Q. *Do I need nose clips?*
A. If you feel uncomfortable exhaling through your nose while submerging, nose clips will help. However, practice exhaling through your nose while bobbing. Soon it will become more comfortable, and you may not need nose clips.

Spas and W.E.T.s

Q. *What are the general benefits of spas?*
A. Besides the other benefits of water, spas add the following advantage: The spa jets massage the body. Massage is known to promote healing of injuries by increasing blood circulation, which increases the oxygen and waste product exchange in

the body tissues. This allows the byproducts of inflammation to be removed more quickly. In addition, the pressure of the water massage helps reduce swelling.

Q. *What safety precautions should you be aware of when using a spa?*
A. Read the signs posted at the spa. If you have an illness or a health condition such as pregnancy, do not use the spa. Also, with the foaming water you may not see a step or may lose your balance. In rare cases, bacterial infections can be contracted from sitting on bench areas close to spas.

Q. *How long should I stay in a spa?*
A. If the water temperature is 104° F (40° C) do not remain in the tub for longer than 15 minutes.

Q. *Why such a short time?*
A. High water temperature can raise the body's temperature and the temperature of your internal organs beyond safe limits—it would be similar to having a fever. If you wish to remain in the spa for longer than 15 minutes, you may:
   1. lower the temperature of the water to body temperature, 98.6° F, or
   2. leave the spa after 15 minutes, take a shower, cool down, and return.

Q. *What are recent developments in spa technology?*
A. Over the last 25 to 30 years the spa has progressed from a single-jet whirlpool tub to a sophisticated hydrotherapeutic apparatus with clustered jets for the back, neck, shoulders, and feet. The jets move in a pattern to bring progressive relaxation to targeted muscle groups. In addition, special air injections are available for whole-body therapy. Many of today's spas are made of state-of-the-art Lucite, which is available in a wide range of shapes and colors, and is easy to maintain. The average spa is eight feet in diameter, holds four to six people, and is filled with about 400 gallons of water (weight: 3,000 pounds). In North America, such a spa could cost from $1,000 to $3,500.

Q. *Can I do exercises in a spa?*
A. Yes, a spa is ideal for doing warm-ups and simple stretches. However, don't overdo it, and don't stay in the spa for longer than 15 minutes.

Q. *Can young children use a spa?*
A. Yes, but they need supervision, and they need instruction on how to enter and how to leave the spa. They should know that spas are not made for jumping, diving, or for swimming underwater. Never let kids use the spa unsupervised. For children, the temperature of the water in the spa or hot tub should be close to body temperature.

Safety and W.E.T.s

Q. *What safety precautions should I be aware of around water?*
A. In a pool, look before you plunge! Check for water clarity, depth, other bathers, safety equipment, diving boards, and for lifeguards on duty. Remember: Never swim alone.

   In open-water areas, check for posted precautions, including water temperature, currents, tides, submerged pilings, etc. Never dive into unknown waters. Learn rescue breathing and cardiopulmonary resuscitation (CPR) by taking a course offered by your local American Red Cross or American Heart Association chapter.

Q. *What are the basic safety skills to learn?*
A. Knowing cardio-pulmonary resuscitation is a lifesaver. ABC refers to three crucial points in an emergency situation.
   A = Airway: Make sure that the victim's airway is unobstructed.
   B = Breathing: Check to see that the victim is breathing, by noting movement of the chest cavity.
   C = Circulation: Check for pulse. If properly trained in CPR, start chest compression if no pulse is found, in order to maintain blood supply to the brain.

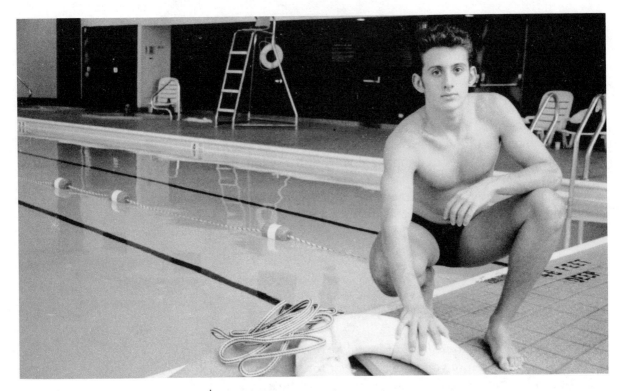

If you own a pool, it is best to be thoroughly trained in CPR. Contact your local Red Cross chapter or the American National Red Cross.

Q. *Does swimming pool water make you more susceptible to infections?*

A. Pool water is chemically treated and filtered continuously for your safety and comfort. The key to keeping your body less susceptible to infection is to dry off properly after your workout. (There is always a fungus among us!) If you are susceptible to athlete's foot or jock itch, be certain to dry these areas thoroughly, and use a powder or cream made for either of these problems. Women will find that water does not enter the vagina because of the overlapping of the anterior and posterior walls. Be certain before you plunge into the pool to check the odor, clarity, and cleanliness of the water. If the pool has a chronic "ring around the collar," you may want to look for another facility.

HYDRATE—WATER IS BEST!

Although it is easy to take water for granted, water is the body's most important nutrient. We can survive only a few days without it, and it comprises 60% of our total body weight. It is a solvent for digestion, helps to lubricate joints, helps to regulate body temperature and helps rid the body of waste products. Because the body's metabolism is increased during exercise, replacing water lost during workouts is important. This includes water workouts; it is easier to forget to hydrate because you are surrounded by water, because even though you may feel like it's "no sweat" to do your W.E.T. workout, you do sweat!

One suggestion is to have a handy water bottle available poolside. If not, remember to hydrate before and after your W.E.T. workout.

Distilled Water: Water which has been evaporated into steam and then recondensed. Technically it is the purest because all solid matter has been eliminated; however, because there are no minerals or sodium, it tastes flat.

Mineral Water: This is water, usually from a spring, which contains some minerals. "Natural" mineral water has all the minerals that were in it when it was taken from the ground.

Seltzer Water: This is tap water which has been filtered and carbonated, without added minerals or salts. Flavored seltzers usually have the essence of fruit juice mixed in (one tenth of one percent).

Sparkling Water: This is a generic term for any type of carbonated water. These usually contain sodium.

Club Soda: This is filtered tap water which is carbonated and to which minerals/mineral salts are added. The taste of each brand comes from the specific combination. These generally contain sodium also.

Spring Water: Spring water must come from a source that naturally arises from the ground, with or without processing. "Natural spring water" must be bottled directly at the source.

Q. *After my W.E.T. workouts, I get thirsty. What should I drink?*

A. Water! It is an essential nutrient with zero calories that will replenish your internal water supply after exercise. It's best to drink cool water, which will enter the bloodstream at a faster rate. Remember, even though you're in water and so can't see any sweat, you *are* perspiring. So replenish your vital water supply with H_2O.

Rx and W.E.T.s

Q. *I've recently recovered from a bone fracture. When can I do W.E.T.s?*

A. As soon as you get permission from your doctor to start bearing weight again. Begin your W.E.T.s slowly. Use the relaxed variations of your W.E.T.s and then move to more difficult levels. Do not overdo it; progress slowly and comfortably.

Q. *I'm a weekend athlete. Can W.E.T. workouts help my aches and pains?*

A. Simulate your sport activity with your W.E.T. workouts. The more energetically you can exercise against the water's resistance, the more conditioning and strength you'll obtain.

Q. *I have a chronic back (knee, shoulder, etc.) condition; can W.E.T. workouts help?*

A. First, check with your physician. Then, choose the W.E.T.s that are comfortable for you. Remember that the massaging effect of water, especially the forceful jet of a whirlpool or spa, helps to increase circulation in the affected area.

Q. *Can the W.E.T. workouts help me relax after my tennis match, round of golf, etc.?*

A. Yes, the massaging and relaxing effects of the water (especially warm water) will help ease those land-made aches and pains.

Q. *I have a heart condition; are W.E.T. workouts good for me?*

A. When you get your doctor's okay to exercise, begin your W.E.T. workouts slowly and do the relaxed versions. W.E.T.

workouts are a good alternative to terra-firma activities, even if you are not a swimmer.

Research and W.E.T.s

Q. *What are the cardiovascular benefits of Water Exercise Techniques vs. fitness swimming?*

A. Recent research has been done comparing the aerobic benefits of water exercise to those of swimming. In this study at John Jay College of the City University of New York, aerobic fitness was measured by the important goal of a slower resting heart rate at the end of the program. There were 55 participants who were within an age range of 19 to 35 years.

  As a result of participating in water exercise classes twice weekly for 8 consecutive weeks, improvements in resting heart were observed. These improvements were comparable to the heart rate of those who participated in traditional lap fitness swimming during the same period. A practical advantage to water exercise is that it requires no swimming ability to obtain the same benefits.

  More recently, researchers from Temple University have shown that working out in water is an effective exercise regimen, and does not jar the joints. Twenty participants, all older adults, were divided into two groups; one group exercised in the water 40 minutes for three days a week while the other group remained inactive. After 12 weeks, those who exercised had improved their aerobic capacity by 15% over the group that remained sedentary.

Q. *What does research say about length of time in a spa?*

A. Recent studies have recommended that sitting in a spa or hot tub for 15 minutes in 104° F temperature is sufficient. After that, your body is telling you to get out so you don't overheat. More and more, health centers and spa resorts are utilizing the benefits of water in their facilities.

Q. *What are recent developments in water exercise?*
A. *Watsu*, meaning water shiatsu, is a relaxing therapy technique both physically and psychologically. Originating primarily in Japan and originally based in Harbon Springs, California, it involves a one-on-one technique of being cradled and moving through the water in a non-threatening, comfortable manner.

Appendix—Sources of Aquatic Information

Suppliers/Manufacturers

AARDVARK SWIM AND SPORT
14101 Sullyfield Cr. #220
Chantilly, VA 22021
(800) 729-1577

AFA, Inc.
aquarobics™
Box 5752
Greenville, SC 29606
(864) 877-8428

AQUA JOGGER
Excel Sports Science, Inc.
450 West 5th Avenue
Eugene, OR 97401
(800) 922-9544

AQUAsource International
5508 North Rockwell
Bethany, OK 73008-2051
(800) 728-4157

AQUATICA
515 Seabreeze Blvd.
Suite 1000
Fort Lauderdale, FL 33316-1623
(305) 922-1899
http://www.aquatica.com

ARENA, N.A.
6900 South Peoria Street
Englewood, CO 80112
(800) 685-6988

BARRACUDA SPORTS PRODUCTS
Skyline Northwest Corp.
0224 S.W. Hamilton Street
Portland, OR 97201
(800) 547-8664

BIOENERGETICS
200 Industrial Drive
Birmingham, AL 35211
(800) 433-2627

B-WISE ENTERPRISES, INC.
109 Possum Way Ct.
Clarks Summit, PA 18411-5958
(800) 360-WISE

COMPETITIVE AQUATIC SUPPLY
15131 Triton Lane
Suite 110
Huntington Beach, CA 92649
(800) 421-5192

COMPETITOR SWIM PRODUCTS
910 Lake Road
Medina, OH 44256
(216) 725-4997
74677.2364@compuserve.com

D.K. DOUGLAS CO., INC.
299 Bliss Road
Longmeadow, MA 01106
(800) 334-9070

DOLPHIN INTERNATIONAL CORP.
Catherine and Sterley Streets
P.O. Box 98
Shillington, PA 19607
(800) 441-0818
[monofins]

FINALS SWIMWEAR
1466 Broadway, Suite #500
New York, NY 10036
(800) 345-3485

FLOATING SWIMWEAR, INC.
P.O. Box 30
Derby, KS 67037
(800) 374-8111
fsiwear@aol.com

FORCE FINS
715 Kimball Avenue
Santa Barbara, CA 93103
(800) FIN-SWIM

GULBENKIAN SWIM, INC.
70 Memorial Plaza
Pleasantville, NY 10570
(800) 431-2586
(914) 747-3240 NY

H₂O WORKS
585 Slawin Court
Mt. Prospect, IL 60056
(800) 323-5999

HIND CORPORATION
3765 South Higuera
San Luis Obispo, CA 93401
(800) 235-4150
(805) 544-8555 CA, HI, and AK

**HYDRO-FIT AQUATIC
FITNESS GEAR**
1328 West Second Avenue
Eugene, OR 97402
(800) 346-7295

**HYDRO-TONE FITNESS
SYSTEMS**
16691 Gothard Street,
Suite M
Huntington Beach, CA 92647
(800) 622-8663

**INT'L SWIMMING HALL
OF FAME MAIL ORDER
COMPANY**
5755 Powerline Road
Ft. Lauderdale, FL 33309-2074
(800) 431-9111
horner@swimstuff.com

**J & B FOAM
FABRICATORS, INC.**
P.O. Box 144
Ludington, MI 49431
(800) 621-3626

**JD PENCE AQUATIC
SUPPLY**
3139 Pacific Avenue
Forest Grove, OR 97116
(800) 547-2520

KIEFER INC.
1700 Kiefer Drive
Zion, IL 60099
(800) 323-4071

**LESLIE'S SWIM & POOL
SUPPLIES**
20222 Plummer Street
Chatsworth, CA 91311
(800) 233-8063

LINCOLN EQUIPMENT, INC.
2051 Commerce Avenue
Concord, CA 94520
(800) 223-5450
lincoln@ix.netcom.com

METRO SWIM SHOP
1221 Valley Road
Stirling, NJ 07980
(800) 526-8788
metswim@ix.netcom.com

NIKE SWIMWEAR
P.O. Box 5959
Portland, OR 97228
(800) 828-2393

NorCal SWIM SHOP
2449 2nd Street
Napa, CA 94559
(800) 752-SWIM

POLAR HEART MONITOR
99 Seaview Boulevard
Port Washington, NY 11058
(800) 743-9248

RECREONICS, INC.
4200 Schmitt Avenue
Louisville, KY 40213
(800) 428-3254
aquatics@recreonics.com

RYKA, INC.
555 S. Henderson Road
King of Prussia, PA 19404
(800) 255-7952

**SPEEDO® AUTHENTIC
FITNESS™ CORP**
6040 Bandini Blvd.
Los Angeles, CA 90040
(800) 5-SPEEDO
(800) 547-8770

**SPRINT ROTHHAMMER
INTERNATIONAL**
P.O. Box 3840
San Luis Obispo, CA 93403
(800) 235-2156

SPORTWIDE, INC.
P.O. Box 16134
San Luis Obispo, CA 93406
(800) 631-9684

SWIMSKIN
675 Forest Avenue
Portland, ME 04103
(800) 341-0246

SWIM ZONE
918 4th Street North
St. Petersburg, FL 33701
(800) 329-0013

THE VICTOR
2725 West 81st Street
Hialeah, FL 33016
(800) 356-5132
swim@victor.net

**TRU-WEST SPORTS
PRODUCTS**
P.O. Box 1855
Huntington Beach, CA 92649
(800) 322-3669

TURBO, INC.
216 Oxford Hills Drive
Chapel Hill, NC 27514
(800) 484-8557 x 1664
turboswim@aol.com

TYR SPORT
P.O. Box 1930
15391 Springdale Avenue
Huntington Beach, CA 92649
(800) 252-7878

**WATERMARK TRAINING
EQUIPMENT, INC.**
2801 Academy Drive, Suite "A"
Auburn, WA 98092
(800) 939-5510

WATERWEAR
P.O. Box 687
Wilton, NH 03086
(800) 321-7848
h20wear@aol.com

ZURA SPORTS
975 Eastwind Drive, Suite 150
Westerville, OH 43081
(800) 890-3009

Publications/Aquatic Magazines

**AQUATICS
INTERNATIONAL
MAGAZINE**
Intertech Publishing
6151 Powers Ferry Road N.W.
Atlanta, GA 30339
(770) 618-0278

**FITNESS SWIMMER
MAGAZINE**
c/o Rodale Publications
P.O. Box 7421
Red Oak, IA 51591
(800) 846-0086

POOL AND SPA NEWS
Leisure Publications
3923 West 6th Street
Los Angeles, CA 90020
(213) 385-3926
psn@pool-spanews.com

SPORTS PUBLICATIONS, INC.
(Publishers of: *Swim* magazine,
Swimming World magazine, and
Swim Technique magazine)
228 Nevada Street
El Segundo, CA 90245
(800) 345-7945

TRIATHLETE
121 Second Street
San Francisco, CA 94105
(800) 441-1666
http://www.triathletemag.com

USA TRIATHLON
P.O. Box 15820
Colorado Springs, CO 80935-5820
(719) 597-9090
trifedusa@aol.com

**WORLD AQUATIC NEWS
AND TRAVEL**
P.O. Box 70366
Pasadena, CA 91117
(818) 793-2582

General Aquatic and Related Organizations

AAHPERD
1900 Association Drive
Reston, VA 22091
(703) 476-3400

AMERICAN COUNCIL ON EXERCISE
P.O. Box 910449
San Diego, CA 92191
(800) 234-9229

AMERICAN NATIONAL RED CROSS
8111 Gatehouse Road
Falls Church, VA 22042
(703) 206-7180

AMERICAN PHYSICAL THERAPY ASSOCIATION
1111 Fairfax Street
Alexandria, VA 22314
(703) 684-2782

ARTHRITIS FOUNDATION, NATIONAL OFFICE
1330 West Peachtree Street
Atlanta, GA 30309
(800) 283-7800

AQUATIC EXERCISE ASSOCIATION
P.O. Box 1609
Nokomis, FL 34274
(941) 486-8600

AQUATIC THERAPY AND REHAB INSTITUTE
1032 So. Spring Street
Port Washington, WI 53074
(414) 284-3633

COUNCIL FOR NATIONAL COOPERATION IN AQUATICS
P.O. Box 26268
Indianapolis, IN 46226
(317) 546-5108

DISABLED SPORTS U.S.A.
451 Hungerford Drive
Suite 100
Rockville, MD 20850
(301) 217-0960

INTERNATIONAL HEALTH RACQUET AND SPORTS CLUB INFORMATION
253 Summer Street
Boston, MA 02210
(800) 228-4772

INTERNATIONAL SWIMMING HALL OF FAME
(Headquarters and Museum)
1 Hall of Fame Drive
Fort Lauderdale, FL 33316
(305) 462-6536

JEWISH COMMUNITY CENTER ASSOCIATION
15 East 26th Street
New York, NY 10010
(212) 532-4949

NATIONAL RECREATION AND PARK ASSOCIATION
Aquatics Section
650 West Higgins
Hoffman Estates, IL 60195
(847) 843-7529

NATIONAL SAFETY COUNCIL
1121 Spring Lake Drive
Itasca, IL 60143-3201
(800) 621-7615
http://www.nsc.org/nsc

NATIONAL SPA AND POOL INSTITUTE
2111 Eisenhower Avenue
Alexandria, VA 22314
(703) 838-0083

PARALYMPIC CONGRESS
1201 W. Peachtree Street
Atlanta, GA 30309
(404) 875-9380

**PRESIDENT'S COUNCIL
ON PHYSICAL FITNESS
AND SPORTS**
701 Pennsylvania Avenue N.W.
Suite 250
Washington, DC 20004
(202) 272-3421

SPECIAL OLYMPICS
1325 G Street, N.W.
Washington, DC 20005
(202) 628-3630

**U.S. MASTERS
SWIMMING, INC.**
2 Peters Avenue
Rutland, MA 01543
(508) 886-6631
75677.2433@compuserve.com

**UNITED STATES WATER
FITNESS ASSOCIATION**
P.O. Box 3279
Boynton Beach, FL 33424
(407) 732-9908
uswfa@pbfreenet.seflin.lib.fl.us

**WORLD WATERPARK
ASSOCIATION**
P.O. Box 14826
Lanexa, KS 66285-4826
(903) 599-0300

YMCA OF THE U.S.A.
101 N. Wacker Drive
Chicago, IL 60606
(800) USA-YMCA

YWCA OF THE U.S.A.
726 Broadway
New York, NY 10003
(212) 614-2700

Special Needs

ARJO, INC.
8130 Lehigh Avenue
Morton Grove, IL 60053
(800) 323-1245

AQUACISER, INC.
Underwater treadmill
5036 Gore Circle
Vail, CO 81657
(800) 825-8798

AQUATIC ACCESS, INC.
Water power lifts, etc.
417 Dorsey Way
Louisville, KY 40223
(800) 325-LIFT

AQUAT TRENDS, INC.
Water Workout Station
649 U.S. Highway One, Suite 14
North Palm Beach, FL 33408
(800) 296-5496

**ENDLESS POOLS SWIMMING
MACHINES, INC.**
200 East Dutton's Mill Road
Aston, PA 19104
(800) 732-8660
http://www.endlesspools.com

**HORTON SAFE-LIFT
HORTON PRODUCTS
COMPANY**
P.O. Box 36277
Pensacola, FL 32516
(800) SAF-LIFT

ICI ACRYLICS, INC.
P.O. Box 15391
Wilmington, DE 19850
(800) 253-8881

REHAB SYSTEMS
Swim-Step™ Pool Access System
1720 Third Avenue No.
Fargo, ND 58102
(800) 726-8620
ndplastic@ad.com

SPECTRUM POOL ACCESS
Lifts and safety ladders, ramps
7100 Spectrum Lane
Missoula, MT 59802
(800) 776-5309

Health and Nutrition Sources

**AMERICAN COLLEGE OF
SPORTS MEDICINE**
P.O. Box 1440
Indianapolis, IN 46026-1440
(317) 637-9200

**AMERICAN HEART
ASSOCIATION**
7272 Greenville Avenue
Dallas, TX 75231
(800) 242-8721
http://www.amheart.org

**AMERICAN MEDICAL
ASSOCIATION**
515 North State Street
Chicago, IL 60610
(312) 464-5000

W.E.T. WORKOUT LOG

Comments:

WARM-UP
(5 min.)

_____   _____
_____   _____
_____   _____

W.E.T. SET   **Upper:** _____   _____
(10–30 min.)   _____   _____
                           _____   _____

Middle: _____   _____
           _____   _____
           _____   _____

Lower: _____   _____
          _____   _____
          _____   _____

Total: _____   _____
          _____   _____
          _____   _____

COOL-DOWN   _____   _____
(5 min.)   _____   _____
                  _____   _____

CHARTING YOUR W.E.T. WORKOUT: PERSONAL W.E.T. LOG

			MAIN W.E.T. SET							
Month	Week	Day	Warm-Up	Upper	Middle	Lower	Combination	Cool Down	Total	Comments e.g., THR
1	1									
	2									
	3									
	4									
2	5									
	6									
	7									
	8									
3	9									
	10									
	11									
	12									

Complete W.E.T. List

Warm-Up/Cool-Down
Aqua Lunge
Arm Stretch
Ballet Leg Stretch
Cross Chest Stretch
Head Circles
Leg Split
Overhead Stretch
Pike Body Stretch
Runner's Calf Stretch
Runner's Quadriceps
    Stretch
Shoulder Shrug
Standing Tall
Toe Tester
Triceps Stretch
Water Walking

Upper Body
Arm and Wrist Swirls
Hang "10"
Medley of Strokes
Push-Ups
Rear Push-Ups
Scull and Hug
Sculling
Sport Arm Pump
Sport Swings (and Follow-
    Through)
Water Push

Middle Body
Back Extension
Body Wave
Buttock Squeeze
Circle Spray
Hip Touch
Knee Tuck
Corner Leg Swing
Overhead Sway
Sit-Ups
Trunk Twist

Lower Body
Aqua Dancer
Aqua-Jog
Leg Crossover
Leg Lunge
Leg Swirl
Leg Treading
Medley of Kicks
Plié Squeeze
Rockette Kick
Side Swipe
Wall Walk

Total Body/
    Combination
Aqua Jumping Jacks
Ballet V
Coordinated Sport Arm
    and Leg Motions
Create Your Own Stroke
Crossover Toe Touch
The Freestyler
    (The Backstroker,
    The Breaststroker,
    The Sidestroker,
    The Butterflyer)
Pendulum Body Swing
Treading
Tug-of-War

Equipment Exercises
Arm Scull and Clap
Barbell Curls
Breaststroke Swim with
    Log (Noodle)
Cossack Kick
Deep Water Jumping
    Jacks
Deep Water Sit-Ups
Hamstring/Thigh
    Challenge

Helicopter
Kickboard Presses (Kick-
    board Waterfall)
Paddle Sports Swing
Paddle Planes
Quadriceps Stretch
Rocking Horse Leap
Side Swipe
Sit 'n' Kick with Fins
Stepping
Workout Station Stretch

Sport Exercises
Aquatic Step Challenge
Archery
Basketball Jump for
    Height
Boxing Punches
Cross-Country Skiing
Dance Leg Lift
Deep Water Running
Diving Approach: Three
    Steps and Hurdle
Double Board Press
Downhill Ski Moguls
Football
Gymnastic/Ice Skating
    Arabesque
Hurdles
Roller Blading
Soccer Kick
Sports Swing
Volleyball Spike
Weightlifting Triceps Kick-
    board Press

Swim Drills/Skills
Alternating Backward
    Arm Circles
Apple Picking
Aqua Jumping Jacks
Backward Jump Rope

Bobbing with Breathing
Body Wave
Breathe with Head Turn
Butterfly Lunge
Butterfly Stroke with
    Single-Beat Kick
Double Arm Circles
Elbow Lift Stroke Cheek
Face Float and Recovery
Flutter Leg Motion and
    Coordination
Forward Jump Rope
Karate Kick
Marching Leg Steps
Paddle Scull
Scissors Lunge
Scratch and Stretch
Splashback
Stroke and Breathe
Treading Arm Scull
    Motion
Treading Bicycle Leg
    Motion
Windmill Arm Motion
Windmill Backstroke

Strengthening
Alternate Toe Touch
Arm and Shoulder Deck
    Stretch
Calf Stretch
Flexibility Stretch
Helicopter
Hip Flexor
Horizontal Water Walk
Knee Lift
Lateral Neck Flexion and
    Extension
Shin Curls

Arthritis/ Special Needs
Figure-Eight Movements
Hand and Foot Small
    Motor Movements
Mastectomy Exercise
Relaxation Float

Pregnancy
Back Massage
Calf Stretch (Ladder/Stair)
Effleurage
Pelvic Tilt
Posture Check

Swing and Sway
Water Kegel

Synchronized Swimming
Bent-Knee Marching Step
Clam
Marlin Turn
Shark Circle
Tuck Turn

Spa
Footsies
Spa Sit 'n' Kick

Spa Sit 'n' Stretch
V Victory Stretch

Pool
Dancer's Leg Stretch
Lateral Ladder Stretch

Beach and Open Water
Sand Jog
Crabwalk
Sandy Sit-Ups
Surfer's Arm Paddle
Leg Sand Sweeps

Family
ABC
Kickboard Sit
Porpoise Dive

Partner
Double Water Wheel
Kickboard Press
Kickboard Race
Partner Hamstring
    Stretch
Partner Quadriceps
    Stretch

Index

About the Author

Jane Katz, Ed.D., is a World Masters champion swimmer as well as an educator, author, and lecturer on aquatics and other aspects of health and physical fitness. She has been a consultant to the President's Council on Physical Fitness.

Dr. Katz is a professor of physical education at John Jay College of Criminal Justice. She is the author of *Swimming for Total Fitness*, *Water Fitness During Your Pregnancy*, and *The All American Aquatic Handbook*.

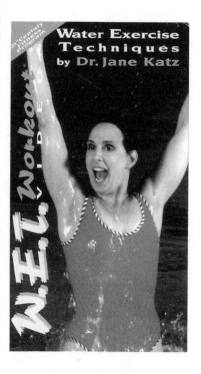